AF824174

Growing Young

THE SEVEN DECISIONS THAT CAN DRAMATICALLY INCREASE YOUR HEALTH SPAN & LIFE SPAN

ALSO BY DR. RON LEE DAVIS:

Choosing Joy: The Pathway to a Life of Passion and Purpose

Ten Traits of a Healthy Parent

Healing Life's Hurts

Gold in the Making

Mentoring: The Strategy of the Master

Courage to Begin Again

A Forgiving God in an Unforgiving World

Mistreated

Becoming a Whole Person in a Broken World

A Time for Compassion

Growing Young

THE SEVEN DECISIONS THAT CAN DRAMATICALLY INCREASE YOUR HEALTH SPAN AND LIFE SPAN

DR. RON LEE DAVIS

amazon publishing

Published by: Independent Publishing

Published in the United States of America

ISBN: 978-0-578-33323-6

DEDICATION:

To my five precious grandchildren.

Having the honor of sharing my life's journey with each of you motivates me to do my part every day to seek to become more spiritually, emotionally, and physically healthy.

The cover photo captures the author and four of his grandchildren enjoying an evening jog together on a Santa Barbara beach.

Photo by Stacy Madden

CONTENTS

PROLOGUE

My beloved mother died peacefully one evening as she was approaching her 95th birthday. It was on the Friday after Mother's Day. Every Mother's Day, I sang a song to mom that I had learned in our church choir as a boy. On this Mother's Day, mom's final one on earth, I sang the song to her one last time. One verse contains these lyrics:

"May I remember each day
To show my love in some way.
Oh, may God bless you and keep you,
Keep you, mother dear."

Our loving God answered the prayer found in these lines. Mom was spiritually, emotionally, relationally and cognitively vital until the final moments of her life. In the morning of her final day, she told me she felt fatigued and wondered if she might be coming down with a cold. After a nap in the afternoon, she awoke to compliment a friend on her beautiful new blouse, and serenely fell back to sleep — never to awaken.

Decades of research have led me to this conclusion: many more of us ought to be dying after a long and full life in the manner of my beautiful, kind and compassionate mother. Overwhelming psychological, sociological, nutritional and kinesiological data indicate that there are seven essential decisions we must make if we are to age in a healthy and vital manner. The seven decisions are to:

1. **Decide to develop and maintain a strong bond of love with family and friends.**
2. **Decide to develop and maintain a life of meaningful service to others.**
3. **Decide to develop and maintain a life of consistent exercise primarily in nature.**
4. **Decide to develop and maintain a plan for lifelong brain health.**
5. **Decide to commit yourself to fueling your body with excellent nutrition.**
6. **Decide to create an ideal environment for restorative sleep and other experiences of rest and renewal.**
7. **Decide to develop a plan which will enable you to grow spiritually throughout all the seasons of life.**

For many years, I have sought to live and teach others this foundational life principle: what we pray for, we give ourselves to! For example, if I pray for the welfare of poor and needy families in my community, I must also, in some way, give myself to help and support these friends in need. If I pray for restored harmony in a broken relationship between two friends, I must seek to be available as an agent of reconciliation to enable healing and restoration. In the same way, if I pray for a long and healthy life that is well lived in service to others, I must give myself *fully* to this goal. Achieving a long health span and life span are endeavors we pursue in partnership with God. We must daily do our part by the decisions we make.

The San Antonio Spurs have been one of the most consistently successful basketball teams in all of professional basketball over the past twenty years. Inside the Spurs locker room, there can be found only one quotation. It is engraved on a large plaque and reads:

> *"When nothing seems to help, I go and look at a stonecutter hammering away at his rock perhaps a hundred times with-*

out as much as a crack showing in it. Yet, at the hundred and first blow, it will split in two, and I know it was not that blow that did it — but all that had gone before."

Jacob Riis

Many of the practical suggestions found throughout the pages of this book may feel challenging to you. Yet if you apply them with the diligence of the stonecutter, these recommendations will ultimately yield a healthier, longer and more meaningful life.

Before sunrise every morning, as a part of my quiet time of prayer and meditation, I ask myself this penetrating question: *"What can I do today that I will be grateful for doing five years from today?"* Then, I briefly touch a bracelet I wear that reads simply, "I must". It reminds me that today ***I must*** seek to follow the seven decisions of healthy aging as I do my part, in partnership with God, to live a long and healthy life in service to others.

My mother used to say to me periodically, "I want to die young as late as possible." My prayer is that you, as you read this book, might come to experience an even greater health span and life span as you grow younger each year until one day you peacefully pass into eternity. The practical guidance and most current research related to the seven crucial decisions shared in the pages ahead can serve as a guide for you to achieve this worthy goal.

❖

The First Decision

"The heart that loves is always young."
Greek Proverb

"A sweet friendship refreshes the soul."
Proverbs 27:9

The First Decision

DECIDE TO DEVELOP AND MAINTAIN STRONG BONDS OF LOVE WITH FAMILY AND FRIENDS

In the 1950's, the small town of Roseto, Pennsylvania raised considerable interest in the scientific community because of its strikingly low rate of premature deaths. Epidemiologists began to carefully study the citizens of Roseto, expecting to discover very low levels of major health risk factors: cigarette smoking, a sedentary lifestyle, obesity, poor nutritional choices. To their great surprise, the Rosetans' health habits were no better than those of other Americans. Rather, the protective factor for the citizens of Roseto appeared to be the intimate social fabric of the community.

The extended family was vital in this homogeneous Italian-American community in the 1950's. The citizens of Roseto were not highly mobile in this period of their history. Extended family members and friends knew one another intimately, their joys and sorrows. Many of the two-story stone homes in Roseto were filled with three or even four generational families who attended church services together every Sunday. Neighbors wandered in and out of one another's kitchens regularly, and holidays were joyously celebrated with loved ones together.

Sadly, by the 1960's, as Roseto became more Americanized and less close-knit, the rate of premature deaths rose to the national level. However, after a fifty-year study, the original researchers concluded that close family ties and a cohesive network of friendships in the 1950's turned out to be *the most important factor* in predicting the health span and life span of the citizens of Roseto.

Thirty years of research lead me to the inescapable conclusion that if we choose to live the typical American lifestyle, we are unlikely to reach our potential maximum lifespan. In fact, it is likely that we may fall short of living a healthy and energetic lifestyle by a decade or more if we fail to honor the seven decisions outlined in this book. And none of the seven decisions is more important than the first one — *to develop and maintain strong bonds of love with family and friends.*

Here are four important truths that we now know about the relationship between a long and healthy life — and a strong social network.

1. Isolation is a powerful risk factor for both poor health and premature death.
2. Social support from family and friends in its many forms has a direct positive effect on health and longevity.
3. People without two or three close friends have five times the likelihood of premature death.
4. The most common factor among known centenarians is the presence of strong social

bonds, deeply rooted relationships and the unconditional love shared with their families and friends and/or faith communities.

Throughout this book, I will frequently refer to the "blue zones" — the five communities in the world with the longest living men and women (Sardinia, Italy; Okinawa, Japan; Loma Linda, California; the Nicoya Peninsula of Costa Rica; and Ikavia, Greece).

A pivotal characteristic in these five diverse communities is a passionate commitment to family and to the development of deep friendships. Dan Buettner, the leading research scientist regarding the sociological patterns of the citizens of the "blue zones" writes:

"The most successful centenarians we met in the blue zones put their families and friends first. This commitment is perhaps the most powerful decision you can make to extend the quality and length of your life. For example, the residents of Loma Linda, California are predominately Seventh-day Adventists who make a point of associating

consistently with one another, a practice reinforced by the observation of a weekly family-oriented Sabbath."

THE BLUE ZONES

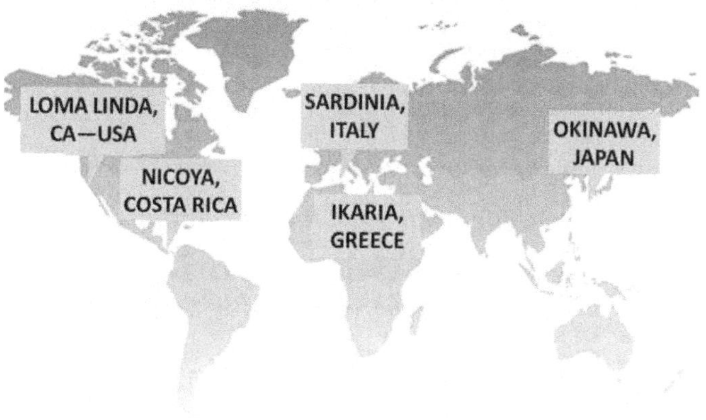

The residents of the five communities in the "blue zones" deeply believe that there is nothing more important for their health span and life span than the quality of their human relationships. Scientific research is affirming the conviction of these villagers. Dr. Dean Ornish, the pioneer physician who first demonstrated the link between diet and the reversal of heart disease, reviewed all the existing scientific literature on the link between loving relationships and our health. He then wrote the groundbreaking book *Love and Survival*. In it he writes:

> *"I am not aware of any other factor — not diet, not smoking, not exercise, not stress, not genetics, not drugs, not surgery — that has a greater impact on our quality of life, incidence of illness, and premature death than the priority of loving relationships.*
>
> *I have summarized literally hundreds of studies showing that people who feel lonely and isolated are many times more likely to die prematurely than those who are closely bonded with family and friends, not only from coronary heart disease, but from virtually all causes of premature death. We sometimes can view the time we spend forging out friendships as luxuries that we do only after the important stuff in our lives is done. Yet, research makes it clear that this* **is** *the 'important stuff.'"*

Dr. Ornish is not the only esteemed medical icon to become convinced of the healing power of our relationships with one another. Dr. David Spiegel, professor of Psychiatry and Behavioral Sciences at Stanford Medical School, told the annual meeting of the American Psychiatric Association of the surprising results of a study he had conducted. Dr. Spiegel and his colleagues had been studying eighty-six women with metastatic breast cancer. The women had been randomly placed in two groups. Both groups received the same medical treatment, but one group also attended weekly support group meetings. To the amazement of the researchers, the ten-year study found that the women who participated in the support group had nearly *twice* the survival rate of the women in the control group. Spiegel later told the Los Angeles Times that the women in the support group not only lived nearly twice as long, but they also experienced fewer mood swings and less pain than their counterparts. These gains clearly came from the loving relationships built during the 90-minute weekly sessions, during which women were encouraged to express whatever they were feeling, including fear, anger, depression, guilt or anxiety. The women who participated the most actively in the meetings experienced the greatest lengthening in survival time. Although all of the women in the study had been labeled as "terminal", all of the women in the support group were still alive when Spiegel made his presentation *twelve years* after the study began.

Could Dr. Spiegel's study have been an aberration? A few years later, Dr. F.I. Fawzy and his colleagues at the University of California at Los Angeles Medical School conducted a study similar to Spiegel's, this one dealing with the survival rates from malignant melanoma in two groups of patients. As in Spiegel's study, the patients in both groups received the same medical treatments and were equivalent at the beginning of the study in terms of the degree to which their cancer had progressed. The only difference was that one group also met regularly for mutual support. Five years later, the researchers were stunned to find that individuals in the group that did not participate in the support group were *three times* more likely to have died than those who had the opportunity to build loving relationships where they could talk through their experiences.

In a similar study, psychologists from Brigham Young University examined the habits and social connections of more than three hundred thousand participants and found that a lack of strong relationships increases the risk of premature death from all causes by 50 percent. A Harvard University publication notes that this lack of relationship building through social connections is roughly equivalent in health effects to that of smoking fifteen cigarettes a day.

The value of authentic intimacy to our health span and life span is difficult to overstate. The British Medical Journal conducted a study that further demonstrates this reality. For seven years, they followed 752 men. At the onset of the study, these men had been given a medical exam during which they were asked about their emotional stress. The study found that those men who had reported being under serious emotional stress at the time of their initial exam had more than triple the risk of dying during the seven years following the exam. Being under these kinds of stresses at the beginning of the study turned out to be a stronger predictor of dying within the ensuing seven years than medical indicators such as high blood pressure, high concentrations of blood triglycerides or high cholesterol levels. What made this study astounding was that for the men who said at the outset of the study that they had a committed web of intimacy and love through close friends and/or family, there turned out to be *no correlation whatsoever between high stress levels and death rate.*

What this study, and a myriad of scientific research projects like it, tells us is that loving relationships have an extraordinary ability to defuse the negative medical effects of stress. Clearly, our connections with the significant people in our lives, if they are positive, affirming and loving, can prevent stress-induced illness, greatly contribute to our health and healing, and add many years to our lives. These scientific studies corroborate what we've learned about the citizens of the "blue zones" — that their abundance of meaningful, loving relationships is one of the primary secrets of the world's healthiest and most long-lived peoples.

Professor Lisa Berkman of Harvard University has devoted her life to investigating the relationship between social connectedness and longevity. In her study, she observed the impact of close social ties with family, faith communities and the ability to develop and maintain deep, authentic friendships. The results of her research over a period of nearly a decade demonstrated a dynamic and vital relationship between loving bonds of friendship and physical health. Those with the least social connectedness were between two and three times more likely to die during a nine-year period than those with the most social connectedness. One recent meta-analysis initiated by the U.S. Council on Aging concluded:

> *"Social isolation and loneliness are clearly associated with increased mortality. Social isolation has also been linked to other adverse health effects, including dementia and increased risk for hospital admission from all causes."*

Much of the content of this book was written during the worldwide COVID-19 pandemic. It became apparent to me in the early months of this tragic plague that the term "*social distancing*" was a misnomer. To be sure, we must practice *physical distancing* to help stop the spread of COVID-19, but socially, many of us may emerge from this crisis feeling closer to our family and friends than ever before.

Each day brings new examples of deepening bonds with loved ones as the pandemic continues. In Italy, neighbors isolated in their homes found shared comfort by singing in unison from their windows. In Canada, communities organized teams to ensure groceries were delivered weekly to the ill and elderly. In my community, the drive-in theatre re-opened, and every week I'd pile my grandchildren into the car for a family-friendly movie with each vehicle parked at least six feet apart from the next car. Friends shared with me that when loved ones were hospitalized with a no admittance policy, they would gather outside the window of the hospital room to wave and to pray for their sick family member. I participated in Zoom appointments where I reconnected with friends whom I had not seen in many years. As we learned to play and work and collaborate in new ways, we were helping each other fend off isolation, and reminding each other just how vital strong bonds of love are for our emotional and physical health.

Multiple studies verify that from birth we need the touch of love from others. My daughter, Rachael was born eleven weeks prematurely. She weighed only three pounds at birth, and within a few days her weight dropped even further. Soon, Rachael's breathing became labored. Our team of physicians determined that, as a consequence of being born almost three months prematurely, she had contracted hyaline membrane disease, a serious respiratory distress. From the hospital where she was born, she was rushed by ambulance to Children's Hospital in downtown Minneapolis. There she was placed in a tiny incubator, with orders from our medical team that she was to remain in isolation for one full year.

I was aware of research that indicated that the stroking touch of love on the arms and legs of a premature baby could contribute to the healing process. My wife and I vowed to spend several hours every day and evening stroking her through the tiny holes in the sides of the incubator. Finally, after one year, Rachael was diagnosed as completely healed and allowed to interact with other babies, family members and friends. Our pediatric radiologist later told me that he had never read of a baby born so prematurely, with so many diverse lung infections, who had lived.

During my visits to be with Rachael, I came to know another young couple whose baby was born prematurely with similar lung diseases. The pain of watching their precious little one covered with tubes and a respirator became so difficult for them that they stopped coming to visit their baby regularly. Soon after, the infant passed away.

No one can know for certain if these parents' lack of connection contributed to the death of their child they loved so deeply. However, we do know there is a phenomenon referred to as the "Failure to Thrive Syndrome" that demonstrates a clear correlation between physical touch and a baby's health and well-being.

For several years, I travelled annually overseas to provide hunger relief and agricultural development in famine-stricken countries. Feeding and holding many malnourished babies, I was often reminded of words I had read years before by Edmund Janss:

> *"In Madras, India, I once watched a house mother tenderly holding a baby. She was feeding her while humming a gentle song. The baby had been found in a trash heap softly crying. I asked the house mother about her feeding method. She nodded and said, 'If we don't hold them and stroke them, and touch them as we feed them, the babies die. But if we hold them and stroke them and touch them as we feed them, they generally live."*

Contemporary psychological and sociological studies confirm the ancient truth of Ecclesiastes 4:9-10:

> *"Two are better than one, because they have a good return for their labor. If either of them falls down, one can help the other up. But pity anyone who falls and has no one to help them up."*

Researchers have identified three circles of relationships that are necessary for emotional and physical health. The first circle is filled with an intimate partner. This could be your spouse, your best friend, or your closest confidante. Tucked away in I Samuel 18:1 is the beautiful verse that reads, "David loved Jonathan and their souls were knit together." It is this kindred spirit relationship that fills the first circle. The second circle is filled by close friends. These friendships are affirming, vulnerable and loyal. I include my two adult children in this second circle of relationships as they are both close and beloved friends to me. The third circle is filled by relationships in our communities. I so enjoy interacting daily with the college students who work at a nearby coffee shop, kind and loving members of my faith community and friends of my family whom I may stop and chat with at the grocery store or a local restaurant. All three circles of relationships are necessary for our physical and emotional well-being, and I regularly do a self-evaluation to discern how committed I am to be nurturing all three circles.

The reality that people with a great deal of social support are healthier and tend to live longer is no longer debated. The psychological and sociological data is overwhelming. But the ever-recurring question that follows is: Why? What is it about developing and maintaining a strong social network that is health promoting?

In the broadest sense, the answer to this question is that God has created us to be in deep, authentic, loving relationships with one another. When people aged 60 and over are asked what specifically they need from their social network, they respond with these types of support:

1. Someone to confide in about the challenges and joys of life.

2. Someone to reassure them of their love and support.

3. Someone to demonstrate respect and affection.

4. Someone to talk with about their health concerns or about life struggles.

5. Someone to provide care when illness strikes.

Throughout my life, I have found these various types of support not only from my family, but through my commitment to meeting regularly in support and accountability groups. For example, for over 16 years while living in the Bay Area of California, I was part of a men's support/accountability group led by my friend Dave Barry. Dave describes the impact of our group with these words:

> *"It was amazing to me that a group of men, each in the midst of busy careers, agreed to meet weekly to support and pray for one another. The accountability piece was developed over time. First, we had to learn to trust one another. Most of the men did not know each other well, if at all. From the start we all agreed that everything said in the group was to stay in the group. It is one thing to say this; over several years we came to believe it. Developing relationships based on honesty and trust allowed us to be vulnerable. We regularly asked the other men to hold us accountable and followed up with each other weekly to see how we were*

doing. Often what one person was struggling with, another man in the group had dealt with as well, and we were able to help and encourage each other. We prayed for each other at the close of the weekly meeting and prayed throughout the week seeking God's guidance and direction for our lives.

It seemed that there was never a time that at least one of us was not going through something difficult and challenging. The accountability group was there to help each other deal with serious illness, death, job loss, addiction issues, wayward children, divorce, legal issues, and so forth.

Several of the men in the group became my closest friends. I know if I had an issue at 3 a.m. they would answer the phone and be there for me — and I would do the same for them. I praise God for putting our group together and blessing us with friendships and support that endures to this day, even though many of us moved throughout the country."

In 2019, I was diagnosed with prostate cancer. I immediately sought out support from family and friends. My son and daughter-in-law, Nathan and Emily; and my daughter and son-in-law, Rachael and Justin were all wise and compassionate in their loving guidance. They accompanied me to doctor's appointments, offered insights as I weighed various treatment options and stood by me as I faced MRI's, CT scans, biopsies and weeks of radiation therapy. In addition to their support, I invited a number of my friends to become a part of my "Healing Team." These loved ones prayed for me daily and regularly checked upon my emotional, spiritual, and physical well-being. I consulted with five physicians whom I knew and trusted, including my life-long friend, Dr. Bill Richardson. I felt inspired by the support of my social network and often reflect on what a difference these family members and friends made through this season of my life. The radiation treatments proved successful.

The first of the seven decisions reflected on in this book has often been a challenging commitment for me to make. I am temperamentally an introvert and enjoy prolonged periods of solitude and study. Yet, I have come to believe deeply that the quality of my social network will be crucial for me in the years to come, and I block out time daily for meaningful, authentic, vulnerable sharing with my family and friends. The importance of a vital social network to successful aging cannot be overstated. So may it be an essential characteristic of all our lives.

❖

The Second Decision

"I slept and dreamt that life was joy.
I awoke and saw that life was service.
I acted and behold, service was joy."
Rabindranath Tagore

"The greatest among you will be a servant."
Jesus Christ, Matthew 23:11

The Second Decision

DECIDE TO DEVELOP AND MAINTAIN A LIFE OF MEANINGFUL SERVICE TO OTHERS

Over a dozen years ago, I made one of the best decisions of my life. I decided to move from the Bay Area in northern California to Santa Barbara in order to be near my daughter, son-in-law, and their children. At the time, Rachael and Justin had two children, with a third baby on the way. I arrived in Santa Barbara on the day that Cami was born, and three years later, grandchild number four, Griffin, was conceived.

In moving to Santa Barbara, I was hopeful that I could be of some practical help to my family and invest my life in my four grandchildren. With

Rachael's and Justin's enthusiastic support, I have been able to do this — and it has brought tremendous meaning into my life.

Not every person can live near their family, but research is clearly indicating to us that we all need to discover a life of meaning and service to others. In the "blue zones" those five communities described earlier in this book, the world's longest living peoples do not refer to "retirement" at all — but continue to live lives of active service to others into their 80s, 90s and beyond.

Epidemiologists indicate that an essential characteristic of men and women who live long and healthy lives is "the necessity of feeling necessary." Further, we know that a deep sense of experiencing meaningful service to others acts as a buffer against stress and depression, as well as reducing the likelihood of our suffering from dementia, arthritis, stroke and other diseases as we age.

Dr. Robert Butler and his collaborators led a National Institute of Health funded study that observed the correlation between having a strong sense of purpose and longevity. His 11-year study followed highly functioning people between the ages of 65 and 92 and found that individuals who expressed a clear goal in their life related to serving others lived longer lives and were significantly more mentally acute than those who did not have a strong life purpose. Dr. Dorothy Height observed:

> *"Without service to others, we will not have a strong quality of life. It is important to the person who serves as well as the recipient. It is the way in which we continue to grow and develop throughout life."*

Dr. Walter Bontz, clinical professor of Medicine at Stanford University writes: *"The life affirming and life extending power of having a defining sense of purpose related to service to others is the intangible factor that is incalculable in value."* Investing in your relationship with loved ones with a servant heart will have profound health and life extending impact.

Psychologist and gerontologist Dr. Ken Dychtwald writes wisely when he states:

> *"There is nothing more important to our daily well-being as we age than to have a*

clear sense of purpose for our future. When I turn eighty-eight, ninety-two or ninety-seven, I may have some regrets. But those regrets won't include spending too little time with my family or pursuing a life I didn't feel passionate about, or failing to seek to serve the needs of others."

Psychologist Erik Erikson, the father of adult development theories, writes wisely when he states, *"I am what survives of me."* American philosopher William James echoed Erickson's words when he wrote, *"The great use of life is to spend it for something that will outlast it."* I'm often guided by the philosophy of German author, sociologist and psychoanalyst Erich Fromm, when he wrote:

"*Giving is the highest expression of true power. This experience fills me with joy. Giving is more joyous than receiving, not because it is a deprivation, but because in the act of giving lies the expression of my aliveness."*

To understand how crucial it is for us to clearly define our sense of purpose as we age, it is helpful to gain some historical perspective. Just 160 years ago the elderly were a tiny fraction of the world population. Less than 5 percent of Americans and Europeans reached aged 65 in 1860. The figure remained well below 10 percent as recently as 1930. Now, projections have the number of 65 year olds globally doubling by 2050, at which time there will be more people over age 50 than under age 15, and the average 50 year old will be able to expect to live another 40-plus years. I live by the philosophy that if we are not going to die soon, we are not old. If we are not old and may have many years left on earth, it is crucial for us to be very intentional and focused upon our goals and objectives in this season of life.

Over the decades of my life and ministry, I've always admired people who come into my life who are reinventing themselves as middle aged or older adults. The mother who enrolled in law school at age 45, motivated to become a defense attorney for the poor. The widowed couple in their 80s who asked me to officiate at their wedding as they have fallen in love and yearn to commit their lives to each other. The retiree who starts a whole new career after his retirement stage begins to become boring. The friend who goes back to college and receives her doctorate in Educational Psychology at age 70. The fellow runner who challenges me to train with him for his first marathon at age 62. These are men and women who understand the words of scholar Joseph Campbell, *"We must be willing to rid ourselves of the life we've planned so as to have the life that is waiting for us."*

One of my great heroes is Dietrich Bonhoeffer, the German Christian martyr and theologian who wrote from prison these words: *"A righteous person is one who lives for the next generation."*

I've long kept those words on my nightstand and am reminded of them each evening and morning. As I look back on my life, the most meaningful moments have come from experiences like:

- Traveling to Third World countries to aid in hunger relief and agricultural development

- Camping with inner-city children each summer for several years

- Teaching a friend who had experienced a stroke how to read again

- Studying together with many young men in one-on-one weekly sessions discussing passages of Scripture or a quality book such as The Seven Habits of Highly Effective People by Stephen Covey

- Teaching my son how to shoot lay-ups on our backyard basketball court

- Feeding the homeless on Wednesday evenings at a neighborhood park

- Planning weekly "dates" with each of my four grandchildren

While I can never know what impact these activities had on others, I am deeply aware of the meaning these experiences have had on my life. And we know now that a life marked by service to others will enhance the possibility of our living long and healthy lives. My friend, Bob Kraning, Director of Forest Home Christian Camping Center for many years, wrote these words before his death in 2020:

"The ultimate success of my life will not be judged by the number of those who admire me for my accomplishments, but by those who attribute their wholeness to my love for them — by the number of those who have seen their true beauty and worth in my eyes."

One mentor of mine who lived by these words was Ken Heileger. Ken began investing in my life when I was eight years old and continued to positively impact my life until his death. Ken was my Sunday School teacher in fourth, fifth and sixth grades. Throughout my junior high and high school years, Ken never missed a sporting event or choir concert in which I or one of his other students participated. He was a tremendous model of Christian love.

Ken had such an impact on my life that I asked him to speak at both my ordination and installation services. When my brother died at age 41 from cancer, our family asked Ken to speak at his funeral. Ken and his wife, Ann, never had children of their own, but in a very authentic way, they had hundreds of children. I used to walk through their kitchen and noticed dozens of photos taped onto their walls and the refrigerator — photos of adults Ken and Ann had mentored and loved since childhood. While other professional men and women may have diplomas and recognition plaques on their office walls, Ken's office was filled with pictures of men and women to whom he had given his time and energy and oftentimes had helped financially obtain a college education.

Throughout the decade of his seventies Ken continued to invest in my life and the lives of others. When he passed away, I wept and spoke at his memorial service to a standing-room-only crowd — a life well-lived by a man who found meaning and purpose by investing his life in children and teenagers.

My friend Don Nason made a significant decision in his mid-60's that has added great meaning and purpose to his life over the past fifteen years. He writes:

"I am told that being happily retired can be difficult. However, in my case I have developed interests out-

side my technical profession to build on, so cultivating new passions was not a problem for me. One particular activity has been a highlight. I volunteer in inmate rehabilitation activities in the California Prison System. The program is called Alternatives to Violence, and I have been involved in it for 15 years.

I organize and facilitate workshops for inmates who spend three days doing group activities that build their skills in non-violent communication, team building and self-awareness. It has been very fulfilling in important ways:

- *I believe it's God's work because it's spiritually significant for the inmates and myself. The eagerness of many inmates to atone for, and recover from, acknowledged misdeeds and estranged relationships is thrilling to see.*

- *I like challenges, autonomy and some calculated risk-taking. Making the logistics work in an environment originally designed for confinement and inmate control, not rehabilitation, can be a challenge. I enjoy inventing useful, new activities.*

- *I have found great satisfaction in involving inmates*

in facilitating the program. I challenge and trust them, which helps their rehabilitation and builds leadership skills useful to their eventual release.

- *After a hesitant beginning, my wife is now fully involved so we can share the experiences, enriching our lives together.*

Neither my wife nor I have ever felt endangered by inmates. Outside volunteers are greatly appreciated by inmates for volunteering their time to bring programs which help inmates prepare for and qualify for release back into society. As many inmates have told us: 'If something goes down around here, you are the ones we would be protecting'. This is nice to hear, and it is reinforced continually by the general goodwill of inmates who appreciate that such programs are available.

Perhaps the most enjoyable thing about our prison ministry life has been the relationships we develop with participating inmates. This is based on the blessing of being able to view them for what they want to be, not for their crime or what they want to leave behind. This is Second Chance Thinking. It's a blessing to be able to maintain this viewpoint and act on it.

It is difficult to overstate the role that meaningful service to others plays in healthy aging. Often, this role is filled by the simple act of volunteering. Allan Luks, Executive Director of Big Brothers Big Sisters and author of the book "*The Healing Power of Doing Good*", surveyed three thousand adult volunteers, and discovered that 95% of them reported a "helper's high" or feelings of energy and euphoria while serving others. Many noticed they were suffering fewer aches and pains and even a reduction in the frequency of the common cold. Similarly, a study by the University of Michigan discovered that men and women ages 65 and above who volunteered lived significantly longer than those who chose not to be involved in service to others. In a comprehensive review of existing data, the Corporation for National and Community Service concluded that volunteers have greater longevity, higher functional ability, lower rates of depression and less incidents of heart disease.

"There is now a convergence of research leading to the conclusion that helping others makes people happier and healthier", writes Dr. Stephen Post, a professor at Case Western Reserve University

School of Medicine and coauthor of "*Why Good Things Happen to Good People: The Exciting New Research that Proves the Link Between Doing Good & Living a Longer, Healthier, Happier Life.*" Dr. Thomas Sanders, Executive Director of the Saguero Seminar at Harvard University, puts it this way, "*Meaningful service to others is the new hybrid health club for the twenty-first century as we age.*"

Over the past five decades, I have been invited to help a number of my friends prepare to transition from their careers into their retirement years. My goal is always to help each person discover a deeper and richer life in this season of their pilgrimage than they have ever experienced before. So often people are trained to think of their skills and talents as what they do for their vocation or career. But if we can think of these talents more broadly and see them as core strengths, then we discover our skillsets are much more widely applicable as we dream of the next chapter of our lives.

I always encourage friends to reflect on their primary interests as they prepare for the next chapter of their lives. If a friend wants to approach this exercise in a more systematic manner, I suggest they consult with a career counselor or certified, experienced life coach. Further, I have helped lead friends through online evaluations such as the Myers-Briggs Inventory.

I also ask friends how they spend their discretionary time each week. Most of us tend to be drawn to the settings, activities, groups and friends that allow us to express our interests and utilize our gifts. As we continue to visit together, I ask friends to think about their hobbies and what exactly makes these activities exciting for them. Related questions I raise include:

- What inspires you?
- What are you truly passionate about?
- What do you deeply love doing?
- What most stimulates you?
- What puts you in a state of 'flow'?

These are the kinds of questions that help us focus and understand our life purpose for the next season of our journey. Louis Pasteur once wrote, *"Chance favors the prepared mind."* Yet most people I have known in my life never take the time to involve themselves in this crucial process. Here's a pivotal truth I've observed scores of times in working with people: Because service to others can be demanding and difficult at times, many of my friends don't find true meaning for their lives because they have not connected their gifts with real human needs. Simply put, God has created us in such a way that when we know our talents and link those gifts with authentic areas of need, the result is a joyful life, with huge benefits for our health and longevity.

When I turned 60, I began to consciously and proactively reflect on the question: *"How does God want me to spend this 'third season' of my life?"* Put another way, I asked *"If by God's grace, I live to age 90 or beyond, how can I most impactfully live the next 30 years."* I daily remind myself that I want with intentionality to invest my life in this "third season" in those things that are eternal. I believe the only two things that are truly eternal are:

- Our relationship with God
- Our relationship with people

Accordingly, one of my daily morning prayers is always, *"Loving God, help me today to invest my life in my relationship with You and my relationship with people, because I know everything else will pass away."* So may we all live in this crucial season of life discovering our true purpose as we give of ourselves in loving service to others.

❖

The Third Decision

"If you can't run then walk. If you can't walk, then crawl. But whatever you do, keep moving."

Martin Luther King, Jr.

"Let us run with perseverance the race that is set before us."

Hebrew 12:1

The Third Decision

DECIDE TO DEVELOP AND MAINTAIN A LIFE OF CONSISTENT EXERCISE PRIMARILY IN NATURE

John Altfillisch was a great high school track coach. Under his tutelage, I ran on two state championship cross country teams and helped set the long-standing school record in the two-mile relay at the Drake Relays in 1964. With his quiet, demanding, yet encouraging guidance, I came to develop a life-long love for running. What I did not realize as a high school and college middle distance runner were the scores of benefits far beyond cardiovascular health that can be experienced through consistent exercise.

For example, running, brisk walking and other forms of exercise performed in nature have been shown to be more effective than prescriptive antidepressants in reducing symptoms of mild to moderate depression. A review of twenty-five randomized, controlled trials concluded that "exercise had a large and significant effect on depression, in both mild and moderate depressive disorders." The effects were even stronger if the exercise took place with another individual or a group. Exercise also slows the release of stress hormones such as cortisol, which can help us avoid spikes in feelings of anxiety and fear.

Inhabitants in the "blue zones" don't hold gym memberships or construct weight rooms in their homes. The longest-lived groups in the world tie exercise into the natural movements of their daily lives in nature. They garden or farm their crops. They actively complete their daily chores without modern conveniences. They walk to visit friends at their homes. They hike to their villages when they need supplies. And they tend to live very long and very healthy lives.

In the "Women's Health Study", involving tens of thousands of women, those who walked briskly 30 minutes a day cut their risk of heart attack and stroke in half. In one study of over 55,000 adults, active joggers and runners gained three extra years of life compared with sedentary adults. Further, exercise lengthens our telomeres. Telomeres are the structures at the end of our chromosomes that regulate cellular aging. As our telomeres get shorter, our life potential shortens as well, and the risk of premature death increases correspondingly. People who have consistently high levels of physical activity have significantly longer telomeres than those who have sedentary lifestyles.

Chronic emotional stress can shorten telomeres, but exercise can also prevent this from happening. Those who were sedentary experienced telomere shortening when feeling stressed, but those who exercised daily saw little to no change in telomere length, even if they were stressed.

In one study, adults with high physical activity levels had a biological aging advantage of nine years compared to those who were sedentary, and seven years compared to those who were moderately active. The researchers defined "highly active" as engaging in thirty to sixty minutes of jogging or brisk walking per day, at least five days a week. In other words, exercise has an anti-aging effect at a molecular level.

In another study, scientists researched men and women between the ages of fifty-five and seventy-nine who had been cycling for decades and still pedaled about four hundred miles per month. These adults were biologically younger than their chronological age. Their muscles generally retained their size, fiber composition, and other markers of good health across the decades. The riders who covered the most mileage each month displayed the healthiest muscles, whatever their age. They had an immune system, reflexes, memories, balance and metabolic profiles that more closely resembled those of thirty-year-old's than those of the sedentary older groups.

Psychologists call physical activity that takes place in a natural environment *green exercise*. Within the first five minutes of physical exercise in nature, people report major positive shifts in mood and outlook. The scriptures are filled with references to the wonders of God's creation, and I have long believed that God has created us in such a way that we receive wonderful blessings in so many different ways when we choose a lifestyle that daily causes us to move in nature. I have made this choice for most of my life, and personally affirm the transformational impact of physical movement in the diversity of God's creation. I'm grateful to presently live in Santa Barbara with its picturesque beaches and temperate weather. But even during the thirty years I lived in the often-frigid Midwest, including a decade in Minneapolis, I found ways to join with friends in exercising in nature. Perhaps you are familiar with the old saying, "there's no such thing as bad weather, only bad clothing." In general, I've found the sentiment behind these words to be true and hold in my heart many memories of exercising through cold and snowy winter weather.

Psychologically, we know that simply being in nature increases people's ability to both gain perspective in their lives and to distance themselves from everyday stresses and challenges. At the Hongneung Arboretum in Seoul, Korea, middle aged adults being treated for depression walked among the trees and alpine plants before participating in their weekly cognitive behavioral therapy sessions. At the end of one month, 61% of the forest-walkers were in remission, three times the rate of patients whose psychotherapy took place in a hospital! It is difficult to overstate the psychological value of *green exercise.*

Historically, it is important for us to understand that our tendency to spend most of our days indoors is a relatively recent reversal. Our ancestors spent most of their time outdoors, interacting with nature. Because of this reality, we know that psychologically, the human mind responds to nature in ways that tend to bring out our cognitive strengths and create the potential for us to deeply connect with our Creator. Being in nature daily puts many of us in touch with the innate joy that biologist E.O. Wilson calls *biophilia,* or the love of all that is living and created by God.

A further profound benefit of daily exercise is the impact movement has on the brain. When we consistently exercise, we can literally grow new brain cells. As you may know, this process is called neurogenesis, and we will study this phenomenon more in chapter four. Suffice it to say here that exercise can play a significant part in protecting us from vascular dementia and can enable an aging and shrinking brain to increase in size and can improve memory.

For example, a randomized controlled trial of 120 older adults found that those who were able to walk briskly for forty minutes a day for one year showed brain growth in the hippocampus and, as a result, improvement in their memory and cognitive function. In contrast, the brains in the comparison sedentary group actually shrank.

Another study discovered that men and women with mild cognitive impairment, which is often a precursor to Alzheimer's disease, who exercised four times a week over a six-month period experienced an increase in gray matter volume as measured by an

MRI and showed an improvement in cognitive function. In contrast, the control group who did not exercise showed increased brain atrophy and worsening in cognitive function.

How does this happen? Exercise causes new neurons to be born and also new connections between neurons to be made. This allows us to develop new learning and memory. It also significantly improves our vascular structure in the brain. Beyond increasing the size of our hippocampus, exercise makes the connection between our neurons work more effectively and brings more blood flow to the brain.

Dr. Arthur Kramer, a research psychologist at the university of Illinois writes, *"Exercise is not just a matter of slowing down the aging process. It's a matter of reversing it."* What is the closest we can get to discovering Ponce de Leon's search for the Fountain of Youth? Clearly, it's exercise!

In a 2017 essay, Norwegian ethicist Sigmund Loland posed the question: If it becomes possible, should we replace exercise with a pill? Scientists are already trying to manufacture medicine that mimics the health benefits of exercise. What if they succeed?

"Considering exercise takes time and energy and usually some financial resources in addition to the potential risk of injury, the only reason for not replacing exercise with a pill must be related to values in the very activity of exercising in itself," Loland writes. *"Does exercise have such values, and if so, what are they?"*

Based on my life experience and the research I've dedicated myself to for over three decades, I would answer Loland's question with a resounding yes! Movement in nature offers us meaning, renewal, serenity, identity, belonging, hope and joy. Exercise moves us into places that scientifically we know are good for us, both in the beauty of nature and often in the presence of a supportive community we all deeply need through the seasons of life. Beyond these benefits, it gives to me and to so many I have known throughout life's journey, a unique, transcendent experience with our Creator. Ethicist Sigmund Loland came to a similar conclusion, declaring that an exercise pill would be a poor substitute for physical activity. He writes, *"Rejecting exercise means rejecting significant experiences of being human."*

One form of exercise in nature is referred to as forest bathing. Forest bathing is a Japanese practice of simply walking under a canopy of beautiful trees, immersing ourselves in the wonder of a forest and soaking in the surrounding atmosphere through all our God-given senses. Forest Bathing has been scientifically *proven* to be a way to lower blood pressure and reduce stress hormone production. When we are walking in a forest and breathing in the aroma of the trees, we are also absorbing substances known as phytoncides which can protect us by increasing our natural killer immune cells and decreasing cortisol levels. While spending time in nature has long been recommended to improve emotional well-being, we now understand what the aroma of the forest is doing for both our bodies and brains. We also know that we need not travel to some far-off forest to gain these benefits. For example, several times a week, I walk at a beautiful park near my home surrounded by magnificent trees and flowers for my forest bathing.

Ultimately, I move in nature daily because of the joy it brings into my life. For me, joy is what ties together the neurochemistry of the runner's high, the elation of moving in synchrony, and the wonder of being in God's creation. As philosopher Doug Anderson writes, "The transformative traits of movement in nature are there for each of us if we will awaken to them, if we will pay attention to our own experiences." There is no training formula each of us has to follow. There is no one path or prescription for each of us except to follow our own joy. If we are looking for a guideline, it is simply this: Move. Move whatever parts of your body still move and do it with a heart of gratitude. Move by yourself. Move in community with others. Move to music or an uplifting audiobook. Move in silence. Move. Move — every day for the rest of your life.

One of the most celebrated moments of Olympic history took place at the 1992 games in Barcelona, when British runner and world record holder Derek Redmon finished the 400-meter semifinals dead last. An injury had kept Redmond from competing in the 1988 Olympic games in Seoul, Korea, and so Barcelona was widely considered his last and best chance to win a gold medal. It you have watched the video of the event, you will recall what transpired. Redmond starts strong in the race, but within fifteen seconds, Derek clutches his right leg and slows to a hop. Two seconds later, he collapses onto the track. The violent pain he was experiencing was his hamstring muscle snapping off the bone.

By the time Redmond is able to stand back up, every one of his competitors has crossed the finish line. The race was over. Yet, Redmond refused to quit. He began to courageously hop awkwardly toward the finish line on one leg, grimacing in excruciating pain. Meanwhile, a middle-aged man wearing a baseball cap has sprung from his seat in the stadium and is rushing the track. Officials try to block the man, but he pushes past them. The man reaches Redmond and places a hand on the back of his shoulder. At first Redmond starts to shake it off, thinking it's a race official trying to stop him from finishing the race. Then he hears, "Derek, it's me." Redmond turns to discover that it is his father.

Redmond's father grabs his hand and raps an arm around his son's waist. He jogs alongside his boy until Redmon cries out in pain and slows to a walk. As they take healing steps, Redmond weeps as he buries his face in his father's chest. The two continue to walk around the track. The crowd begins to cheer, and rapidly moves into a massive standing ovation, as Redmond and his father finish the last hundred meters together.

After the event, a Canadian competitor sent Derek a note, calling Redmond's finish, "the purest, most courageous example of grit and determination I have seen."

Redmond's desire to persevere through his pain and finish the race is remarkable. Yet, I personally don't think it's his courage that people are most moved by. Rather, it is his father, the person who didn't belong on the track, but who sprang into action to help his son — he is the one we most remember. This Olympic moment touches us deeper. It brings tears to my eyes each time I watch it. (You can find it on YouTube under the title Father's Day Lookback: Derek Redmond 1992.) For me, this example of a father's love for his boy serves as a metaphor for all those who have come alongside me as I have sought to continue to consistently commit to daily exercise through the peaks and valleys of life. From my high school track coach, to scores of running partners racing 5K races to marathons, to countless basketball games with my children, to beach runs and soccer games with my grandchildren, to walks with friends in nature — we all need each other to continue to move forward through the seasons of life. The closest any of us will come to the elusive fountain of youth is exercise in nature, so let's just keep moving!

❖

The Fourth Decision

"The cultivation of your mind should be the ultimate aim of human existence."
B.R. Ambekar

"Be transformed by the renewal of your mind."
Romans 12:2

The Fourth Decision

DECIDE TO DEVELOP AND MAINTAIN A PLAN FOR LIFELONG BRAIN HEALTH

Over the past three decades, I have spent a great deal of time distilling the best evidence-based brain research. In order to make these scientific discoveries useful and helpful for us, I've created a simple ten question self-inventory assessment to begin our reflections on brain health:

1. Do you avoid strenuous exercise?

2. Are you overweight?

3. Do you sit for most of the day?

4. Do you lack daily social engagement with others?
5. Do you have high blood pressure, diabetes or high cholesterol?
6. Is your diet high in processed, sugary, fatty foods and low in whole grains, nuts, fresh fruits and vegetables?
7. Do you live with high levels of daily emotional stress?
8. Do you have a history of alcohol abuse?
9. Do you experience poor sleep on a regular basis?
10. Do you lack daily cognitive challenges in the form of learning new challenging information?

As you have probably guessed, the more frequently you answer yes to any of these ten questions, the higher your risk becomes of eventually developing mild cognitive impairment, Alzheimer's disease or some other form of dementia. The good news we will discover in this chapter is that changes we make now can often reverse earlier damage we may have done to our brains.

My close friend, Dessiree Searl, age 88, has lost five family members to Alzheimer's disease — including her husband and one of her sons. Yet, despite these tragedies touching her life, Dessiree remains upbeat, positive, joyful. An avid walker who has logged in up to 1,200 miles a year, she serves as volunteer secretary at her church, initiates daily contact with her many friends, pieces together up to thirty complex puzzles a year, eats a healthy diet that keeps her fit and trim, and sleeps peacefully each night. As we will learn from the science-based research in this chapter, Dessiree is making all the correct choices to protect her from the many diseases that fall under the general category of dementia.

Prevention is the most powerful antidote to illness, and this is especially true of the degenerative maladies that can affect the brain. Sadly, well over half of adults in the United States do not know the risk factors for dementia, or the actions that can be taken now to protect the brain.

The Joy of Movement and Brain Health

When I'm asked what the single most important decision is that a person can make to enhance brain health, I respond, *"The research tells us it's one word: exercise."* Exercise is the only behavioral activity *proven* to trigger biological effects that help brain health! As we learned in the previous chapter, we now know that when we exercise, we can literally grow so many new brain cells — called neurogenesis — that our brain can actually get measurably bigger. More importantly, it is the part of the brain that controls memory — called the hippocampus — that gets bigger.

For example, a randomized, controlled trial of 120 older adults found that those who walked for 40 minutes a day for a year had brain growth in the hippocampus and, as a result, improvement in both their memory and their cognitive function. In contrast, the control sedentary group showed growing brain atrophy and worsening of cognitive function.

How does this happen? Science teaches us that exercise causes new neurons to be born, and also new connections between neurons to be made. This allows us to develop new learning and memory. Also of great significance is the reality that exercise protects our vascular structure in the brain. We know that poor vascular flow in the brain causes us to be vulnerable to both strokes and vascular dementia.

The influence of exercise on brain functions is so profound that the American Academy of Neurology recently stated that scientific studies clearly suggest the benefit of exercise for protection from mild cognitive impairment (MCI). Consider that while no particular medication is universally recommended for brain health, *exercise is*!

Dr. Ron Peterson, a physician at The Mayo Clinic and founding member of The Global Council on Brain Health, writes that the field of cognitive development has been revolutionized by imaging technology. PET scans now allow scientists and physicians to look inside the living brain and discover meaningful data. Dr. Peterson goes on to suggest that these advances in technology further affirm that physical activity has the strongest evidence to date of bringing about positive brain changes. In addition to brisk walking, the pioneers in scientific brain research are teaching us that interval training is particularly helpful. Interval training simply means that we alternate between varying levels of speed, intensity and effort. For some, this means moving between periods of leisure walking and brisk walking. For others who are able to do so, this means moving between periods of jogging and sprinting.

I realize the message of the value of exercise has been shared with us all our lives. But what we may not fully realize is the various ways exercise protects our brain health. For example, we now know that both hypertension (high blood pressure) and diabetes significantly increase our risk for dementia later in life. Exercise is a powerful tool to protect us from both these risk factors. Here's a crucial truth for all of us to understand and to lovingly share with our family members: simply being inactive, regardless of our body weight, has been shown to be twice as deadly as being obese. Prolonged sitting has been scientifically proven to dramatically increase our risk for premature death. When we are immobile, our circulation shuts down, and our bodies use less blood sugar, which means more sugar is circulating. Sitting for long periods also negatively influence blood fats, high-density lipoprotein (the good cholesterol), resting blood pressure, and the satiety hormone leptin (which tells us when to stop eating). Further, sitting puts muscles into a dormant state, which can lead to atrophy and muscle weakening. Moreover, when we sit for long periods each day, our metabolic rate plummets and we stop burning as many calories.

Consider a 2018 study which showed that the more fit an older person was, the better the chances he or she could recall words, as compared to those who were less fit. Scientists increasingly believe that exercise can act as a "First Aid Kit" for damaged brain cells, speeding up recovery after injury, stroke or significant emotional stress.

A further profound factor in understanding the relationship between exercise and brain health is related to the issue of stress reduction. When our bodies are experiencing stress, they release the hormone cortisol, which we now know can create long lasting brain changes. Daniela Kaufer, an integrative biologist at the University of California, Berkeley, and her colleagues conducted a series of experiments demonstrating that chronic stress and elevated cortisol levels can negatively affect memory and new learning skills. These scientists discovered that too much cortisol can generate an overproduction of myelin-producing cells and an under-production of neurons. This led to a shrinking of the hippocampus, the memory hub of the brain. However, daily exercise has been shown to minimize the impact of stress and its resulting flood of cortisol.

I hope that the evidence I've shared in this chapter will motivate us to maintain a daily exercise routine of at least brisk walking 40-60 minutes. Dramatic new discoveries are being shared with us every year reflecting the positive relationship between exercise and brain health.

The Power of Purpose and Brain Health

I hope to never retire. I find great meaning and joy in my vocation as a Christian speaker, researcher, author and teacher. I also know the consequences for so many who retire early, including an increased risk of developing dementia. For example, one study showed that for each additional year of meaningful work, the risk of being diagnosed with dementia is reduced by 3.2%. The study, which included nearly half a million people in France, demonstrated that someone who retired at age 65 had a 15% lower risk of developing dementia compared to someone retiring at 60, even after other factors were taken into account. Clearly, staying engaged in meaningful work tends to keep people both socially connected and mentally challenged. In the "blue zones" there isn't even a word for retirement. Aging men and women in these five communities remain socially active in their vocations well into their 80s and 90s. There is great cognitive power in maintaining a sense of meaningful work and in continuing to learn, discover and complete challenging tasks. So, the conclusion we can draw is this: either don't retire if you love your work, or proactively develop a new active life of challenge and growth in retirement.

One of the most startling conclusions in cognitive research has come from comparing different people's brains when they are autopsied. A significant revelation is that while some brains share virtually identical pathology, the individuals examined exhibited very different levels of competency while they were alive. For example, two brains that look equally diseased at autopsy will not necessarily *in any way* reflect how well the persons engaged in their respective lives. The reason for this disparity is often referred to as one's personal "cognitive reserve" or what scientists sometimes refer to as "brain resiliency." Building this reserve or resiliency is rooted in a person's choice of staying actively involved in life through meaningful work and strong social interaction. Furthermore, we know that an important goal in building and sustaining cognitive reserve is to make demands upon our brains through strategizing, learning new information, solving problems, and often by taking on a challenge such as learning a foreign language or a musical instrument. Two of my friends, Dr. Bill Richardson, a retired physician, and Dr. Gene Lucas, retired Executive

Vice Chancellor of The University of California, Santa Barbara, share their experiences with building cognitive reserve.

❖

As a retired family physician, I have paid attention to the scientific evidence regarding activities that help maintain cognitive and physical health. Fortunately for me, many of them are activities that I already enjoy doing. I have always enjoyed bicycling, and now have time for almost daily rides. Often as I fly down a country road on my bike, my spirit soars with wonder and exhilaration. Also, for decades I have enjoyed backpacking, but only had time for trips lasting 3 or 4 nights. Now, in retirement, I have been able to experience the satisfaction of spending almost a month backpacking the 212-mile John Muir Trail in the Sierras of California. In order to be prepared for the backpacking trips, I take time most days for long walks all over town, and the availability of podcasts has meant that I can walk forever without becoming bored. For cognitive health, I was thrilled to discover that learning to play a musical instrument is of similar value to learning a new language; I'm lousy at learning languages but had always planned to return to piano lessons once I retired. I am now seven years into those lessons, and thoroughly enjoy their mental challenge.

I am fortunate that things which I enjoy also enhance my cognitive and physical health, and I wonder if everyone couldn't likewise find that to be the case. Those who find themselves dreading their daily health activities may have simply chosen the wrong activities. Just like I could substitute the piano, which I love, for a foreign language which I don't enjoy, probably most people could go through the list of healthy activities and find ones they eagerly look forward to. Furthermore, involving friends in one's activities helps nurture a healthy social network while providing accountability. Two or three times a week several of us couples get together for yoga classes or bicycle rides, followed by eating out. Through the pleasure of friendship we are further strengthening our minds and bodies.

Dr. Bill Richardson

❖

I recently turned 70. I've been retired now for over 7 years from the University of California Santa Barbara, where I was a professor of engineering for 36 years, spending the last 11 as the Executive Vice Chancellor.

Over time, I had collected the 11 volumes of Will and Ariel Durant's "The Story of Civilization," and set about reading them. But, as I came upon the great books in that reading (the Bible, the Odyssey and the Iliad, Plato, Virgil, Ovid, Dante, Rabelais, Chaucer, Shakespeare, etc.) I'd set Will and Ariel aside and read the great books.

So, here's what I'm now up to these days:

- *After completing the Durant series, I got involved trying to read the top 100 novels on the Modern Library list. I'm about a third of the way through the list.*

- *I've been asked by UC Santa Barbara to chair a*

number of campus committees. Two of them involve planning and constructing new buildings on campus. I like the challenges, I like interacting with excellent staff and faculty on the committees, and it broadens the number of people with whom I have regular contact.

- *I also work exercises into my daily routine: 5 miles on the stationary bike in the morning. This is followed by knee exercises (for my knee replacement 3 years ago) and, depending on the weather, about a 2-3 mile walk around the neighborhood or a nearby lake in the morning or afternoon*

- *I am a member of a Christian church, and currently am serving as the chair of the Board of Deacons. This has turned out to be an especially challenging job as the pandemic forced us to meet outside for over a year as we held all our meetings on Zoom and shared the trials and tribulations of COVID-19. My church family and my interactions with them helped keep me from becoming a hermit during the pandemic.*

- *Finally, the hobby I chose to pursue was to pick up the mandolin and teach myself how to play it, with the help of YouTube and a few beginners song books. The challenge of learning how to play an instrument (each hand doing different tasks), memorize music and words for each song, and sing as well as play is very good for my brain. I really have to concentrate when I'm playing, so I'm in another world when I practice. It would probably be easier with a younger brain and less arthritic thumbs, but the act itself keeps me younger.*

Dr. Gene Lucas

❖

The Need for Sleep and Brain Health

Recent scientific studies have demonstrated that chronic inadequate sleep is strongly linked to a higher risk of dementia. While we will focus on the role of sleep and relaxation in increasing our overall health span and life span in Chapter 6, allow me to share briefly in this chapter about the relationship between sleep and brain health. Dr. Matthew Walker, professor of neuroscience and psychology at the University of California, Berkeley, is among today's pioneering researchers in the power of sleep. In his early writings, he would suggest that sleep is the third pillar of excellent health, alongside diet and exercise. But, given his latest research about how sleep supports brain health, he now teaches that sleep is the single most effective activity we can engage in to reset our brains.

Sleep is essential for consolidating our memories and filing them away for later recall. Furthermore, sleep "cleans up" the hippocampus so that it can take in new information that it then processes. Without adequate sleep, this memory organization cannot happen. More than affecting memory, a sleep deficit prevents us from processing information in general. So not only do we lack an ability to remember clearly when we sleep poorly, we cannot even adequately interpret information that we receive throughout the day.

A 2017 study of 18,000 adults revealed that logging fewer than six hours of sleep a night was associated with a 44% increased risk for those with prediabetic factors being diagnosed with diabetes. This is important information for us to consider in this chapter because of the well-documented relationship between diabetes and brain health. This study, along with many other scientific findings has led some researchers to refer to Alzheimer's disease as a type of diabetes. Clearly, when the body's insulin system is defective and neurons in particular cannot use insulin properly to fuel their metabolism, the stage is set for cognitive decline.

My final observation in this section of the chapter relates to the link between poor sleep and chronic inflammation. A strong body of scientific evidence now shows that lack of sleep raises our levels of inflammation. In fact, even a single night of inadequate sleep can activate inflammatory processes in our bodies.

Among the more recent findings about sleep has been discovering what some scientists call the "washing" effects of sleep on the brain. During sleep, the body clears waste and fluid from tissues through the lymphatic system. Dr. Jeffrey J. Iliff and his team at Oregon Health Sciences University published a description of the brain's self-cleaning function to get rid of waste. Their research ignited a new field of exploration into the drainage pathway that is now referred to as the glymphatic system. A second paper by Dr. Iliff and two colleagues, Dr. Lulu Xie and Dr. Maiken Nedergaard from The Department of Neurosurgery at the University of Rochester, documented that the glymphatic system goes into overdrive at night, suggesting that deep, restorative sleep provides the setting for a cleansing of our brains.

What all these studies — and so many more — are clearly demonstrating is the direct relationship between sleep and the risk of cognitive decline. Sleep is medicine for our brains. May we elevate peaceful sleep to a place of honor as we seek to age with vigor and vital mental acuity.

The Relationship of Excellent Nutrition and Brain Health

We now have significant evidence that shows us that how we fuel our bodies can go a long way toward protecting our brains. For example, Dr. Martha Clare Morris, a professor of epidemiology at Rush University in Chicago and the director of the Rush Institute for Healthy Aging, conducted the following study. She and her colleagues followed over a ten-year period nearly 1,000 people to discover the relationship between nutrition and cognitive decline. One group followed the Standard American Diet (SAD). A second group followed a vegetarian diet high in green, leafy vegetables, beans, whole grains, limited amounts of nuts daily, and fresh fruit. The difference between the two groups ten years later was profound. People who followed the SAD diet had the fastest rate of cognitive decline. Dr. Morris concluded that the second group following the vegetarian diet added approximately seven and a half years of healthy aging, free of significant cognitive decline.

Perhaps you have heard the saying, "What's good for the heart is good for the brain." In many ways, this statement is true. Common conditions influenced by diet such as elevated blood pressure, high cholesterol and diabetes harm *both* the cardiovascular system and cognitive health. Further, we now know recent studies evaluating the incidence of dementia among large groups of people over several decades have demonstrated decreases in dementia occurring simultaneously with improvement in cardiovascular health.

Dr. Sanjay Gupta, professor of neurosurgery at Emory University School of Medicine and Chief

Medical Correspondent for CNN recommends what he calls the SHARP diet for excellent brain health. Using the acronym SHARP, he guides us to:

S: Slash sugar

Alzheimer's disease is increasingly referred to by some scientists as type 3 diabetes, whereby the brain cannot use insulin normally. Gaining control of our blood sugar can equate to supporting our brain health. Multiple meta studies have found that people with high blood sugar levels had a faster rate of cognitive decline than those with normal blood sugar. Further, it is important to note that as we cut back on sugar consumption, we need to consider the sources of our sugar intake. Sugar from a candy bar or pastry is far different from sugar found in fiber containing fruit. Personally, I use the natural sweetener stevia in place of sugar.

H: Hydrate

Research indicates that as we age, our ability to perceive thirst diminishes. This helps us to understand why dehydration is common among men and women as we age. I often say to myself throughout the day, "drink instead of eat" as research indicates we can mistake hunger for thirst. It's important to understand that even moderate amounts of dehydration can sap our energy levels and weaken our brain rhythm.

The link between hydration status and cognitive ability is well-recognized. Dehydration often leads to cognitive confusion as we age, particularly as it relates to short-term memory loss.

In addition to drinking water throughout the day, green and black tea can decrease our risk for cognitive decline. I personally sip tea throughout the day and my hydration levels remain high. Since researchers have found that even moderate dehydration is associated with confusion, disorientation and cognitive deficits, hydrating throughout the day is a crucial component of a brain healthy diet.

A: Add more omega-3 fatty acids to your diet

Perhaps you have read in recent years about the benefits of omega-3 fatty acids for brain health. We know omega-3 fatty acids, found in foods such as nuts, avocados, chia seeds, flaxseeds, pumpkin seeds, and sunflower seeds are beneficial for cognitive function. Unfortunately, the Standard American Diet (SAD) is extremely high in another type of omega — the omega-6 fats, abundant in processed, fried and baked foods. The unfortunate result is that we consume a disproportionate amount of omega 6 fats. While our ancestors consumed omega 6 and omega 3 fats at a ratio of approximately 1:1, today in America, the ratio has jumped anywhere from 12:1 to 25:1 omega-6 to omega-3 acids.

The evidence of the impact of omega-3 fatty acids on brain health is overwhelming, so we need to be certain we are regularly eating nuts, particularly walnuts, avocados, flaxseeds (I put ground flaxseeds daily on my oatmeal), chia seeds and other healthy seeds.

R: Reduce portion size

The research is clear: most of us, as we age, need to reduce portion size. While there are many strategies for accomplishing this goal, perhaps the most effective is intermittent fasting, which I will outline in detail in chapter 6. One of my heroes, Dr. Mark Mattson, has devoted much of his life to studying the link between intermittent fasting and brain health. Dr. Mattson, a professor of neuroscience at Johns Hopkins School of Medicine, and director of the Laboratory of Neuroscience at the National Institute of Aging, has verified the positive relationship between intermittent fasting (fasting 12-16 hours a day, most frequently fasting from dinner until lunch the following day) and improved neural connections in the hippocampus. According to Dr. Mattson, intermittent fasting challenges the brain, forcing it to react by activating adaptive stress responses that help it cope with disease. Further, we now know that when intermittent fasting is done correctly, it can increase the production of brain-derived neurotropic factor (BDNF), a protein that helps protect and strengthen neural connections while also spurring new growth of brain cells. Reducing portions of food consumption through intermittent fasting is easier than you might think — and its brain healthy.

P: Plan ahead

It is difficult to overstate the importance of establishing the correct home environment for the purpose of healthy brain aging. This is particularly true in regard to what foods we decide to have available to us in our home. Planning ahead whenever we grocery shop is crucial. One decision I made many years ago was to never buy in the grocery store any food that was not whole food, plant based. When we plan ahead in this way, we protect ourselves from giving in to a craving for ice cream, processed foods, sugar laden cookies and pastries.

Another way that we can plan ahead is related to times when we are eating out at a restaurant with family or friends. It has become very easy to go online and review ahead of time the menu options of various restaurants. In the past decade, there has been a dramatic increase in the number of restaurants that offer whole food, plant-based options. Planning ahead in this way protects us from impulsively selecting a menu option that is not healthy for our brains.

Why not give the SHARP diet a try? It will prove to enhance your brain health.

As we have discovered in this chapter, a comprehensive plan for brain health will include consistent exercise, meaningful work, cognitive challenge, loving relationships, peaceful sleep and excellent nutrition. May God help us to join in partnership with Him to protect our brains that we might continue to faithfully serve Him with great love.

❖

The Fifth Decision

"The longest-lived people eat a plant-based diet. Nothing they eat has a plastic wrapper or comes out of a box."

Dan Buettner, The Blue Zones

"So whether you eat or drink, or whatever you do, do all to the Glory of God."

1 Corinthians 10:31

The Fifth Decision

COMMIT YOURSELF TO FUELING YOUR BODY WITH EXCELLENT NUTRITION

My beloved brother, Paul, died in 1985 at the age of 41. Paul was an inspirational Christian, a loving husband and father, an outstanding basketball coach and teacher and a wonderful friend to me and to many. Our family continues to miss him deeply and yearns to carry on his legacy of love.

Paul died from cancer which was growing in his colon and had spread into his liver and appendix. His death long ago motivated me to more aggressively research potential nutritional links between the risk of developing cancer and our daily food choices.

Even as long ago as the 1980s, scientific meta-studies were demonstrating a correlation between the consumption of meat and increased cancer risk. Today, over 1,000 separate studies suggest such a link. In the past 30 years, my research has expanded beyond cancer prevention to an understanding of the role our nutritional choices play in the potential development of nearly all diseases. In studying over 100 nutritional and diet books, reviewing countless scientifically based meta-studies and listening to scores of lectures from the most respected nutritional scientists in the world, I have concluded that the acronym for the Standard American Diet (SAD) is an extremely accurate one.

Two thirds of Americans are either overweight or obese. Carrying extra body weight is strongly linked to premature death. Overweight individuals are more likely to die from all causes, including heart disease and cancer. Seventy percent of those with weight problems also have been diagnosed with either hypertension, diabetes, coronary artery disease, cancer or gastro-intestinal diseases. Yet it is crucial to understand that for the vast majority of people, becoming overweight is not caused primarily by *how much* they eat but by *what* they eat. The concept that people get heavy because they consume a high volume of food is a myth. Eating large amounts of the *right* food is a crucial key to a healthy and long life.

I have sought to condense my research into six scientifically verified "food rules". Following these guidelines will increase your likelihood of a long and healthy life.

1. Eat a whole food, plant-based diet.

In Genesis 1:29, we read that the diet in the Garden of Eden was exclusively plant based: *"God said to Adam and Eve, 'I have given you every plant yielding seed which is upon the face of the earth, and every tree with seed in its fruit, this you shall have for your food.'"* Current scientific research overwhelming points us today to the wisdom of this dietary plan. Eating whole foods simply means eating foods as close to their natural forms as possible. A whole food plant-based diet will therefore avoid all processed foods. As Dr. Joel Fuhrman writes, *"The most important thing to remember about food labels is that you should avoid foods that have labels."*

With so many fad diet books on the market it can be very confusing to know what to eat. Fortunately, the overwhelming scientific evidence is now clear! A definitive consensus is emerging that a whole food, plant-based diet is the healthiest way of eating. This diet will be low in bad carbohydrates (white bread, sweets, sugary cereal, fruit juice, sweetened yogurt, white rice, etc.) and bad fats (pastries, muffins, food containing trans fats and saturated fats, cheese, processed snack foods, fried foods, etc.) This diet will be high in good carbohydrates (vegetables, beans, all legumes, brown rice, whole grains, most fruits, oatmeal, etc.) and good fats (avocados, almonds, walnuts, pumpkin seeds, dark chocolate, flax seeds, peanut butter with no added sugar, etc.). Further, this nutritional plan offers plenty of plant-based protein so that disease causing meats can be minimized or eliminated.

Following this plan of nutritional excellence will mean that on a daily basis we choose to consume mostly plants, vegetables, fruits, soy products and a limited number of seeds and nuts. I follow the scientifically verified acronym developed by Dr. Fuhrman after thirty years of research: G-BOMBS. The letters of the acronym stand for: **G**reens, **B**erries, **O**nions, **M**ushrooms, **B**eans and **S**eeds (including nuts). At the end of each week, I look back on the previous seven-day period to ensure I have consumed adequate amounts of these six ingredients of a whole food, plant-based diet.

To commit to this plan of nutritional excellence, we must minimize or eliminate animal protein and replace it with plant-based protein. Over ten years ago, I gave up all animal products as I discovered the incredible benefits of the thousands of protective factors in plant-based foods that have anti-cancer, anti-heart disease and anti-aging properties.

Dr. Neal Barnard, National president of The Committee for Responsible Medicine, writes wisely, "If beef is your idea of 'real food for real people' you'd better live real close to a real good hospital." (Note: It is important for anyone following a whole food plant-based diet to take a quality B-12 supplement daily.)

2. Practice Intermittent Fasting

Intermittent fasting is an eating pattern that cycles between periods of fasting and eating. The most common type of intermittent fasting is eating during an 8-to-10-hour time frame and fasting for a 14–16-hour time frame. For example, I practice a daily 16-hour fast by concluding dinner by 7pm and not having breakfast/brunch until 11 a.m. the following day. My son Nathan, and many of my intermittent fasting friends practice a slightly longer period of daily fasting. The scientifically verified benefits of intermittent fasting include:

a) Intermittent fasting causes major beneficial changes in several crucial hormones that impact aging, potential disease and weight. This is particularly true of insulin. Meta-studies have clearly demonstrated that intermittent fasting has major benefits related to insulin resistance and leads to an impressive reduction in blood sugar levels. This is of particular importance as one of the most frequent diseases associated with aging is type 2 diabetes.

b) It can reduce oxidative stress and inflammation in the body. Oxidative stress is one of the factors that can cause premature aging and many chronic diseases. Several meta-studies have clearly shown that intermittent fasting will enhance the body's resistance to oxidative stress and inflammation.

c) It has been determined to assist in both weight loss and the reduction of visceral fat. When we don't eat for an extended period of time, we can naturally eat less overall. Further, intermittent fasting gives our digestive systems the ability to rest and recover. I have found that the morning pattern of hydrating, stretching, exercising in nature and then having only two meals – brunch/breakfast and dinner to be very beneficial in reducing the impact of aging, gaining increased energy, and in annual improvement of my blood panel markers.

d) It has been scientifically proven to increase heart health. Sadly, heart disease remains the world's biggest killer. Intermittent fasting has been shown to improve numerous risk factors for health disease, including blood pressure, total and LDL/HDL cholesterol, blood triglycerides, inflammatory markers and blood sugar levels.

e) It increases our opportunity to prolong life span and health span. Intermittent fasting, when combined with a nutrient rich diet, has been proven to enhance our potential to increase our life span. The evidence is enormous and irrefutable that calorie restriction through intermittent fasting is beneficial for lifespan potential for most people.

3. Minimize sugar, white flour, white rice, processed foods and other "bad carbohydrates".

Numerous meta-studies clearly demonstrate that a diet with significant amounts of sugar and other "bad carbohydrates" can raise blood pressure and increase chronic inflammation, both of which are pathological pathways to heart disease. Sadly, in the United States, added sugars account for 17% of the total calorie intake of adults. Nutritional scientists demonstrate to us that sugar consumption is a major cause of obesity and can contribute to the development of many chronic diseases. Prolonged high-sugar consumption drives resistance to insulin, a hormone produced by the pancreas that regulates blood sugar levels. Insulin resistance causes blood sugar levels to rise and strongly increases your risk of diabetes.

Further, eating excessive amounts of sugar can increase your risk of certain types of cancer. A study of over 430,000 people found that added sugar consumption was directly associated with an increased risk of esophageal cancer, and cancer of the small intestine. Another meta-study indicated that women who consumed sugar-laden cookies and pastries more than three times a week were 1.5 times more likely to develop endometrial cancer than women who did not.

Perhaps most significantly, we now know that sugar consumption can increase cellular aging and thereby speed up the entire aging process. We learned in the previous chapter that telomeres act as protective caps, preventing chromosomes from either deteriorating or fusing together. As we grow older, telomeres naturally shorten, which causes cells to age and malfunction. Although the shortening of telomeres is a normal part of aging, unhealthy lifestyle choices can speed up this process. Consuming sugar has been clearly demonstrated to accelerate cellular aging.

It is important to clarify that the natural sugars found in fruits, which also contain fiber, are not harmful. Rather, it is the "free sugars" found in sweets, pastries and processed foods that do the damage and speed up the aging process.

Sugar consumption can be lethal. Fortunately, a decision to move to a whole food, plant-based diet will automatically reduce the number of simple sugars in your daily nutritional intake.

4. Consume at least three grams a day of "good fats", the omega 3 fatty acids.

Food high in "good fats" which contain Omega-3 fatty acids include walnuts, pumpkin seeds, avocados, flaxseed, peanuts, chia seeds, brussels sprouts and hemp seeds.

Meta-studies have discovered that Omega-3 fatty acids reduce inflammation, decrease blood triglycerides and lower the risk of dementia. Further studies indicate that 'good fats reduce the risk of heart disease and stroke.

One of the growing health crises of our time is called the metabolic syndrome. The metabolic syndrome is a collection of conditions. It includes visual fat, high blood pressure, insulin resistance, high levels of triglycerides and poor levels of "good" HDL cholesterol levels. It has become a major public health concern because it increases your risk of many other illnesses, including heart disease and diabetes. Omega-3 fatty acids as a consistent part of your diet can improve insulin resistance, reduce inflammation and heart disease risk, and restrict all the diverse elements of metabolic syndrome. I find one easy way to ensure a daily amount of them is to include flaxseed, chia seeds and walnuts in my daily blueberry/banana/spinach and kale smoothie.

5. **Reduce your intake of total fats, especially the "bad fats", such as trans fats, saturated fats and partially hydrogenated fats.**

Three types of fats — saturated fats, hydrogenated fats and trans-fat — have been identified as clearly harmful to our health. Most of the foods that contain these types of fats are solid at room temperature, such as: butter, margarine, shortening and processed foods. Most saturated fats and animal fats, such as beef, pork, lamb, chicken, as well as animal products including milk, cheese and eggs contain "bad fats". Meta-studies have linked "bad fats" to increases in blood cholesterol levels, higher risk of heart disease, and greater vulnerability to many types of cancer. Citizens of the "blue zones" universally eat little or no meat or other animal products.

6. **The following "Daily Dozen", developed after decades of research by nutritional scientist and physician Dr. Michael Greger, are particularly healthy and nutrient rich:**

    1. Beans
    2. Berries
    3. Other fruits
    4. Cruciferous vegetables
    5. Greens
    6. Other vegetables
    7. Flaxseeds
    8. Nuts
    9. Spices
    10. Whole grains
    11. Adequate Hydration
    12. Daily Exercise

Research has demonstrated that within a whole food, plant-based diet, certain food groups have special nutrients not found in abundance elsewhere. For example, cruciferous vegetables (kale, cabbage, broccoli, brussels sprouts, cauliflower, bok choy, garden cress, radishes, turnips, etc.) have particularly strong anti-cancer ingredients. I keep the Daily Dozen list in a prominent place in my home and seek to follow it each day of the week.

Five Myths About Whole Food, Plant-Based Diets

I have long been disappointed that some of my friends have been reluctant to adopt a plant-based diet due to common misconceptions about nutrition. Following are five myths related to a whole food, plant-based diet.

Myth #1: It's difficult to get enough protein on a plant-based diet.

This myth is by far the most common misconception about plant-based diets. Scientific research is unequivocal — we can easily get all the protein we need on a plant-based diet! In fact, it's difficult *not* to! If we are eating an adequate number of calories from a variety of fruits, vegetables, nuts, grains and legumes, it is very hard to not get plenty of protein.

The sad reality is that the vast majority of Americans eat far too much protein. Recent scientific research suggests that up to 97% of American adults consume *more* protein than is necessary for optimum health. Mayo Clinic registered dietitian nutritionist Kristi Wempen writes, "Contrary to all the hype that everyone needs more protein, most Americans get *twice* as much as they need." Too much protein leads to increased risks of heart disease, cancer, kidney function disorders, osteoporosis, liver disease and other chronic conditions.

Protein is essential to good health — including tissue growth and repair, digestion, metabolism, and the production of antibodies to fight infection. When we digest protein, it is broken down into its component amino acids, which our bodies can use for hormones, enzymes and neurotransmitters. Plant-based foods contain three amino acids in various proportions. By eating a diversity of plant-based foods, we can obtain all the necessary amino acids. For instance, legumes (such as beans) are high in lysine but low in tryptophan and methionine. Grains (for example, brown rice) are low in lysine but high in tryptophan and methionine. Therefore, a meal of brown rice and beans provide a complete protein. This is a frequent choice for me.

It should be noted that several studies suggest that many people over age 65 should slightly increase their protein consumption to protect themselves from sarcopenia (a syndrome characterized by progressive and generalized loss of skeletal muscle mass and strength). It is once again important to remember that all of us can consume all the protein we need from plants. For example, spinach contains 50% protein and asparagus contains 44% protein.

Myth #2: Meat makes us stronger.

Having ministered to professional, college, and amateur athletes all my adult life, I know that this is a common misconception. Finally, the scientific word is getting out among elite, world-class athletes that eating a whole food, plant-based diet actually gives them a competitive advantage and even greater strength.

Well-known body builder and former California governor Arnold Schwarzenegger transitioned from eating meat to a whole food, plant-based diet several years ago. He writes, "If they tell you to eat more meat to be strong, don't buy it. As I got older and began to research nutritional studies, I recognized the fact that we don't need to get our protein from meat. So our family moved in the direction of a vegetarian diet. Now, we are doing it the right way and I love a whole food, plant-based diet much more than when I ate meat."

Sprinter Carl Lewis, winner of nine Olympic gold medals, credits a vegan diet for producing his best times on the track. Dave Scott, winner of six Ironman World Championships, finds strength and endurance on a plant-based diet. Rich Roll credits a vegan diet with changing his life and health and fueling him on his way to becoming a world-class ultra-endurance athlete. Defensive tackle DaQuan Jones became a vegan during his playing career with the Tennessee Titans and influenced many of his teammates to join him. Tom Brady, widely considered to be the greatest quarterback of all time, credits his lengthy professional football career to a primarily whole food, plant-based diet. Alex Morgan, 2019 World Cup Soccer Champion, converted to a whole food, plant-based vegan diet in 2017 and credits this decision with her improved play. And the list goes on and on.

Two excellent resources related to this second myth are: *The Plant Based Athlete*, a best-selling book by Matt Frazier and Robert Cheeke, and the outstanding documentary *The Game Changers* available on Netflix.

Myth #3: A low-carb, high protein diet is good for you.

Tragically, a low-carbohydrate, high-protein diet continues to resurface under various names — the Atkins diet, the Paleo Diet, the Ketogenic diet, the Dakar diet, the South Beach Diet, the Zone Diet, etc. What makes these diets so seductive is that they are based on a half-truth. The half-truth upon which we can agree is that Americans do eat too many simple refined ("bad") carbohydrates such as sugar, white flour, white bread, pastries, etc. Because of this reality, if you reduce your consumption of refined carbohydrates, you will likely lose weight.

However, when these diets suggest replacing refined ("bad") carbohydrates with foods such as bacon, sausage, and steak, they go against the clear guidance of scientific research. A far better choice for our health and longevity is to replace the "bad" carbs with “good carbs” such as fruits, vegetables, whole grains, legumes and soy products in their natural unrefined forms.

Objective scientific research clearly demonstrates that the only diet proven to reverse heart disease, to slow, stop or reverse early-stage prostate cancer, and to slow aging by lengthening telomeres is a whole food, plant-based diet very low in both “bad” fats and “bad” refined carbohydrates.

Myth#4: A diet high in carbohydrates leads to obesity.

Every meta-study comes to the same conclusion — vegans who eat no animal protein, weigh less than vegetarians, who eat some animal protein (cheese, for example). Vegetarians weigh less than meat eaters. Complex carbohydrates are not behind the obesity epidemic in the United States. Meat combined with excess calories is the culprit, according to objective scientific studies. Meat disrupts our intestinal bacteria, which leads to weight gain. Most meat comes to the consumer from factory farms and will therefore contain antibiotics, which leads to weight gain. Meat creates inflammation, which leads to weight gain. Our country's obsession with meat creates obesity far more than the consumption of complex carbohydrates.

Myth #5: A high-carbohydrate diet causes diabetes and predisposes you to heart disease.

Complex carbohydrates do not cause diabetes. Meat and other "bad" fats do. Over consumption of meat leads to insulin resistance and rising insulin levels, a syndrome that is the number one precursor to diabetes and is also a major contributor to obesity.

Some of my friends have initially felt a whole food plant-based high complex carbohydrate diet feels extreme. In my discussions with these friends, I often refer to the words of the brilliant scientist and heart surgeon Dr. Caldwell Esselstyn. He writes, "some people think the plant-based whole food diet is extreme. Half a million people a year will have their chests opened up and a vein taken from their leg and sewn into their coronary artery. Some people would call that extreme."

Further, complex carbohydrates do not cause heart disease. Overconsumption of meat is the culprit. Meat raises our bad cholesterol and can clog our arteries. Meat can also provoke a state of inflammation in our bodies which makes us more vulnerable to heart disease.

Finally, what is deeply meaningful to me is the reality that to the degree we transition toward a whole food, plant-based diet, it not only makes a significant difference in our own lives, but also makes a profound difference in the lives of many others around the world. This imbues our dietary choices with meaning beyond ourselves. Many people are surprised to learn that animal agribusiness generates more global warming due to greenhouse gases than all forms of transportation combined. More than half of the U.S. grain and nearly 40% of the world grain is fed to livestock rather than directly to humans, many of whom are presently starving or malnourished. So, to the degree that we choose to eat a plant-based diet, we free tremendous amounts of resources that can benefit many others as well as ourselves. We have enough food in the world to feed everyone if enough people were to eat lower on the food chain. I find it very inspiring and motivating to learn of a growing number of efforts by people of good will to create this transition, and funnel foods directly to starving and malnourished children.

As a Christian, I deeply believe we are called to be good stewards of God's creation. By transitioning to a plant-based diet, we not only support efforts to reduce the dangerous impact factory farms are having on our environment, but also demonstrate compassion toward the animals who experience indescribable cruelty at these concentrated animal feeding operations. Dr. Michael Gregor, M.D., states: *"The most ethical diet just so happens to be the most environmentally sound diet and just so happens to be the healthiest."* John Robbins, author of *The Food Revolution*, writes wisely: *"It is increasingly obvious that environmentally sustainable solutions to world hunger can only emerge as people eat more plants and fewer animal products. To me, it is deeply moving that the same food choices that give us the best chance to eliminate world hunger are also those that take the least toll on the environment, contribute the most to our long-term health, are the safest, and are also, far and away, the most compassionate toward our fellow creatures."* May we be guided by Robbins' words as we make the decision to commit ourselves to a life of nutritional excellence.

❖

The Sixth Decision

"Sleep is the golden chain that binds health and our bodies together."

Thomas Dekker

"When you lie down, you will not be afraid. Your sleep will be sweet."

Proverbs 3:24

The Sixth Decision

DECIDE TO CREATE AN IDEAL ENVIRONMENT FOR RESTORATIVE SLEEP AND OTHER EXPERIENCES OF REST AND RENEWAL

Over twenty years ago, my sleeping patterns had become so erratic and restless that I submitted myself to a 3-month program at the renown Stanford Center for Sleep Disorders. At Stanford University, I not only learned many practical steps to improve my sleep quality but was also educated about the "sleep crisis" we are currently experiencing in our technology-driven culture.

It is of crucial importance for us to understand the many serious consequences of failing to experience restorative sleep. Routinely sleeping less than six hours a night weakens our immune system, increasing our risk for certain types of cancer. Insufficient sleep also appears to be a key lifestyle factor linked to our risk of developing dementia. Further, inadequate sleep disrupts blood sugar levels so profoundly that it can increase our risk of developing diabetes. Inadequate sleep also increases the likelihood of our coronary arteries becoming blocked and brittle, setting us on a potential path toward cardiovascular disease, stroke, and congestive heart failure. We also now know poor sleep contributes to many psychiatric conditions, particularly increased anxiety and depression.

Beyond the many illnesses that are linked to poor sleep, there is the verified link between insomnia and weight gain. Perhaps you have noticed a desire to eat more when you are fatigued. I have. This is no coincidence. Too little sleep has been found to trigger increased levels of the hormone, ghrelin, leading to growing hunger. This makes overeating more likely, added to the reality that we are awake more hours of each day as we battle insomnia.

Both the quality and the amount of sleep we get each night have an astonishing impact on us as we age. Our body does not momentarily press the pause button during sleep. Rather, it's more like a reset button because sleep is a crucial phase of our regeneration. Sufficient sleep keeps us mentally sharp, creative, attentive, and able to process information quickly. Scientific research has convincingly demonstrated that sleep habits ultimately impact how big our appetite is, how fast our metabolism runs, how strong our immune system is, how creative we can be, how effectively we can cope with stress, and how well we can remember things.

It is difficult to overstate the negative impact of the intrusion of technology into our bedroom and sleep patterns. In 2015, neuroscientist Anne-Marie Change and her colleagues showed that light-emitting devices such as laptop computers and e-readers caused people to take longer to fall asleep because of reduced sensations of sleepiness, decreased secretion of the sleep-inducing hormone melatonin, and a later circadian schedule. Light-emitting diodes (LED's) produce blue wave lengths, and these are ubiquitous in televisions, smartphones, computers, and tablets. Clearly, we need to avoid blue light for several hours before bedtime for optimum melatonin production. Sadly, a profound paradox of our present era is this: advances in technology have allowed us to pull back the curtain on what's going on while we sleep, yet technology is also one of the main reasons our relationship to sleep has become so compromised. We must proactively challenge this trend.

Seven Truths We Need to Understand for Restorative Sleep

1. **We need to transform our bedrooms into peaceful sanctuaries.**

When I was participating at the Stanford Center for Sleep Disorders, their mantra was: Cool. Quiet. Dark. We know that the ideal temperature for restorative sleep is between 60- and 67-degrees Fahrenheit. We also know that we need to minimize all light sources in our bedrooms, including technology devices. We need to decide to get rid of anything in our bedrooms that could distract us from restorative sleep. I am continually transforming my bedroom into a sanctuary, with candles and inspirational music available. I honor an evening technology fast, and intentionally set boundaries that will protect me from any potentially conflicted-oriented conversations or emails after 7 p.m.

2. **We must exercise in nature in the morning to improve our restorative sleep at night.**

Nothing has improved my quality of sleep more than morning exercise in nature, and scientific research affirms that value of this exercise/sleep pattern. For example, a recent study from Northwestern University found that daily morning exercise added approximately forty-five minutes of nightly restorative sleep. Further, we now know that early morning exposure to sunlight while exercising stimulates earlier melatonin release and shifts our circadian rhythm forward. As we discovered in chapter three, exercise helps to heal anxiety and depression for many, and this benefit aids in restorative sleep. Exercise such as brisk walking or jogging also provokes a sharp rise in body temperature, followed by a gradual cooling, which mimics the mutual fluctuations of the circadian rhythm, paving the way for deeper sleep. Scientific research is clearly demonstrating the value to waking up to morning sunlight and walking outdoors for at least thirty minutes early in the day. Multiple meta-studies indicate that staying indoors throughout the day negatively impacts sleep quality. Neuroscience teaches us that we are wired to rise early and absorb the rising sun.

3. We Need to Learn to Change our Thoughts About Sleep

Many psychologists refer to how negative sleep thoughts (NST) can have a profound adverse effect on sleep. Examples of NST's are:

- *I must get eight hours of sleep to be effective tomorrow.*
- *I'll feel miserable all day tomorrow if I don't fall asleep soon.*

- *I'm dreading going to bed soon, knowing how poorly I sleep.*
- *I know I can't fall asleep without a glass of wine at bedtime.*
- *I know if I wake up in the middle of the night, I'll never get back to sleep.*

Cognitive Behavioral Therapy, which has been such a powerful healing practice in my life and the lives of so many, guides us in our understanding of NST's (negative sleep thoughts). When NST's occur at bedtime or while we are awakened in the middle of the night, they tend to cause us to feel anxious or frustrated. In turn, these emotions mobilize the stress response, which tends to increase our heart rate, blood pressure, muscle tension and breathing rate (heartbeats per minute.) This stress response then activates our brain's wakefulness system and simultaneously weakens our sleep system.

One reality we can observe from Cognitive Behavior Therapy is the NST's are usually exaggerated, distorted or erroneous. They serve no purpose, except to make it more difficult to sleep. Once we understand NST's and their harmful effect on our sleep, the next step we must take is to have the courage to learn a process called cognitive restructuring. The aim of cognitive restructuring is simple but profound. Research verifies that as we recognize and replace our NST's with more accurate, positive thoughts related to sleep, we will become less anxious and frustrated about our bouts with insomnia. Through learning to reframe our thinking, we can relax and sleep much more restoratively. (The classic, easy-to-read book *Feeling Good* by David D. Burns, M.D. is probably the primary textbook on Cognitive Behavioral Therapy upon which many other books in the same genre are based. I highly recommend it.)

4. We need to establish excellent sleep-promoting habits.

Research verifies that establishing the correct habits and behaviors will strengthen the brain's sleep system and improve our quality of restorative sleep. One very important habit is to establish a sleep schedule and commit to honoring it daily. Although many people shift their sleep habits and schedule on the weekends to make up for a sleep deficit accumulated during the week, we know scientifically that this is an unwise strategy. Such a pattern quickly sabotages a healthy circadian rhythm so crucial for peaceful, deep sleep.

For example, if we stay up later on Friday and Saturday nights to socialize and then sleep in the next morning, we will likely suffer what sleep specialists refer to as “social jet lag”, irregular sleep patterns detrimental to health. One of many reasons to avoid “social jet lag” is related to what we now know about circadian rhythms. Our body temperature rhythm starts to rise in the morning when we get out of bed, become active, hopefully exercise, and allow ourselves to be exposed to sunlight. If we sleep later on the weekends or following a poor night of sleep, we delay the rise in our body temperature rhythm because we delay physical activity and sunlight exposure. If the elevation in our body temperature is delayed by a few hours, the drop in our temperature in the evening will also be delayed by a similar amount of time. Therefore, if we try to go to bed at our normal time, we will generally have difficulty falling asleep because our body temperature will be elevated. Research clearly demonstrates that sleeping later on the weekends is the primary cause of Sunday-night insomnia, even among otherwise good sleepers. Although at times it may seem counter intuitive, an important sleep schedule rule to follow is this: Get out of bed at approximately the same time every morning, including weekends, no matter how little or poorly we have slept.

Circadian rhythm scientists also concur that it is wise as we age to seek to transition from being "night owls" to "morning larks". Sleep research indicates that non-REM (Rapid Eye Movement) sleep tends to dominate sleep cycles in the early part of the night. As night moves closer to dawn, dream-rich REM sleep begins to move to the forefront of our sleep cycle. Although both types of sleep are important and offer separate benefits, non-REM, slow wave sleep is deeper and more restorative than REM sleep. If we are in the habit of staying up too late, we run the risk of minimizing our important non-REM sleep.

Another important sleep-producing habit is to establish meaningful bedtime rituals. These could include deciding not to get into your bed until 30 minutes before sleep time, disconnecting from stimulating tasks such as on our computers or cell phones at least one hour before bedtime, engaging in activities such as taking a warm bath, reading from a book, sipping herbal tea, or listening to soothing music. Remembering that light suppresses the production of melatonin which signals us to sleep, we need to ensure we are taking steps even before we climb in bed to prepare for restorative sleep. In this regard, the National Sleep Foundation advises using low wattage incandescent bulbs in our bedrooms. Dr. Mathias Basner of the University of Pennsylvania echoed this advice. He writes, "Turn off the lights in your bathroom and instead use the light from the hallway while grooming before bed. Bathroom mirror lights can be excessively bright and thus suppress melatonin excretion."

As referred to earlier in this chapter, we know that blue light, given off by our ubiquitous electronic devices is especially good at suppressing melatonin.

We must be mindful of the wisdom of neurologist George Brainard, a circadian-rhythm researcher at Thomas Jefferson University in Philadelphia, when he writes *"Blue-light radiating electronic devices in the evening serve as alert stimulus that will frustrate your body's ability to sleep later. So, when you turn off your computer or iPhone, it doesn't mean that instantly the alerting effects go away. There's an underlying biology that is stimulated."*

When we ignore this fact, says Dr. Dan Siegel, a clinical professor at UCLA, the result can be a vicious cycle: *"People are exposing their eyes to this stream of photons from these objects that basically tell your brain, 'Stay awake! It's not time to go to sleep yet.' So, it's 10 p.m., it's 11 p.m., it's midnight — you're checking for emails, you're looking for texts — those light beams tell your brain, 'Don't secrete melatonin, it's not time to sleep', and you're up at 12:30, 1:00 a.m. checking some more because you're up, so why shouldn't you check? Now, you go to bed at 1, you wake up at 6 because it's time to go to work, that's five hours of sleep."*

A recent survey discovered that 71% of Americans sleep with or next to their smart phones. It is important for us to understand that light, especially blue light, is interpreted by the brain as an anti-sleeping drug or stimulant — something few of us would willingly give ourselves each night before bed. Fortunately, there are some new technologies that help mitigate blue-light exposure. Yet, ultimately the best choice is to gently escort our smart phones out of our bedrooms at least one hour before we fall asleep. As we seek to follow our fifth truth regarding restorative sleep, it is of crucial important to understand that scientific research indicates that people who have the highest emotional investment in their social media lives are also those who report low sleep quality — as well as increased anxiety and depression.

5. **We need to gradually make small changes in our sleep protocol and not become stressed over our rate of progress.**

Best-selling author Louise Hay writes, *"When a child is learning to walk or talk, we encourage him and praise him for every tiny improvement he makes.*

The child beams and eagerly tries to do better. Is this the way you encourage yourself where you are learning something new? Or do you make it harder to learn because you tell yourself you are a failure?'" For those of us who may have neglected the priority of restorative sleep, re-integrating it into our lives is akin to learning a new skill. The key to our success will be discovered in making specific changes and encouraging ourselves along the way.

Changing all our bad habits regarding sleep is not something we can achieve quickly. Rather, making a lasting change requires taking small daily steps toward our goal. For example, some time ago after my initial research on healthy sleep patterns, I decided to gradually move my "in bed, lights out" time up by 1 hour and 15 minutes. (For me, this meant from 11pm to 9:45pm — you may go to bed far earlier than I do.) I decided to gradually make this change in 15-minute increments over a period of six weeks. I also understood this meant altering my evening dinner time, my time for a technology fast to start, and my late afternoon walk. Research clearly indicates that a self-defeating approach to more restorative sleep is to make dramatic changes and then become frustrated over a lack of immediate results. Far better to remain positive and encourage ourselves with changes that can lead us to deeper and more peaceful sleep.

6. **We need to understand that our eating and drinking habits can have a profound impact on our sleep.**

Eating fatty and spicy foods too close to bedtime can cause stomach acid to build up during digestion and disrupt our sleep. Research has indicated that the following foods eaten in the evening may interfere with restorative sleep: avocado, cheese, sauces, peppers, chili, eggs, nuts, pasta, and bananas. We also know caffeine in its' many forms can hinder sleep. Coffee, colas, black tea, and chocolate all contain the stimulant caffeine, and its effect can take eight hours or longer to wear off fully. A general guideline for most of us to follow is to avoid caffeine after lunch. We need to also be mindful of alcohol intake. While alcohol can cause us to feel sleepy, its effects on the body disturb normal sleep cycles and particularly disrupt the restorative REM (Rapid Eye Movement) sleep. Heavy alcohol ingestion can also contribute to impairment of normal breathing patterns at night and can cause us to wake up in the middle of our sleep cycle when the effects of alcohol have worn off.

7. **We need to deepen our lives of prayer, mindfulness, and meditation in order to experience more restorative sleep.**

Scientific research teaches us that the most common nonmedical causes of insomnia are stress and anxiety. This is sometimes referred to as hyperarousal. Here's how those conflicted by chronic insomnia are described in a joint study by Penn State, the University of Athens, and the University of Madrid:

> *"They generally tend to handle stress and anxiety through the internalization of emotions, which leads to emotional arousal. At bedtime, they are characteristically tense, anxious, ruminative about issues associated with health, work, personal affairs, death, etc. Since the emotional arousal causes physiological arousal, they face difficulties in sleep initiation or returning to sleep after awakenings during the night. As*

a result, they develop a 'fear of sleeplessness' which intensifies their emotional arousal perpetuating their insomnia."

In other words, the vicious cycle is that people who can't sleep are often stressed out, and their stress makes it harder to sleep, which gives them another thing to be stressed out about. John Kabat-Zinn, the founder of Mindfulness-Based Stress Reduction writes wisely, *"If you are having a lot of trouble sleeping, your body may be trying to tell you something about the way you are conducting your life. As with all other mind-body symptoms, this message is worth listening to."*

For many of us, the message may be that we have lost a sense of balance in our lives. A life that prioritizes prayer, meditation and mindfulness can restore that balance. USC professor of gerontology Jennifer Ailshire writes, *"If we can't slow down our thoughts and disengage our minds from the daily stress we experience, we have little chance of getting restful sleep.*

> *Strategies for doing this will vary from person to person, but prayer and meditation are good options."*

When I walk into my bedroom, I seek every night to symbolically leave the day, with all its challenges and unfinished tasks behind me. I kneel down on my exercise mat for a time of sleep preparation. I quietly recite the words of Jesus found in John 14:29, *"Peace I leave with you, my peace I give unto you. Do not let your heart be troubled"*. I also often recite Proverbs 3:24, *"When you lie down, you will not be afraid. Your sleep will be sweet."* Next, I offer bedtime prayers of gratitude, thanking God for *specific* experiences I've had that day, and for the precious people who have interacted with me since morning began.

When I awake in the middle of the night with thoughts crowding my mind, I have found deep breathing, praying for loved ones, and meditation to be helpful remedies. Instead of stressing out about how awake I feel and fearing the approaching fatigue of the next day, I lay flat on my back, prop up an extra pillow and reframe my thinking until I truly believe this is a great opportunity for deep, restful breathing, prayer, and relaxing meditation. This practice takes the anxiety out of our wakefulness and adds an extra layer of gratitude to our well-being.

These seven truths have guided and encouraged me on my journey toward a greater experience of restorative sleep. May we all experience the reality of the words of Jesus, *"Come to me, all you who are weary… I will give you rest."* (Matthew 11:28)

❖

The Seventh Decision

"Spiritual maturity is measured by only one test: how much closer to God's loving character have we become."

Elyse Fitzpatrick

"But speaking the truth in love, we are to grow up in every way unto Him who is our head, unto Christ."

Ephesians 4:15

The Seventh Decision

DECIDE TO PROACTIVELY DEVELOP A PLAN TO GROW SPIRITUALLY THORUGHOUT ALL THE SEASONS OF LIFE

Years ago, a friend of mine shared with me a story about a Christian surgeon he knew and admired. As this young surgeon began to grow spiritually, he began to sense that God was leading him to serve as a medical missionary in a poverty-stricken country. The young doctor shared this new calling with his partner at their office in a very affluent area in Southern California. His partner told him that he would be foolish to surrender his lucrative medial practice to become a missionary in some distant land. However, this young surgeon was not deterred in his new calling and pursued both theological and further medical training to honor his commitment.

Several years later, he received his first assignment. He had been ministering in a distant country for about six months when his previous partner flew over to visit him. On the day of his partner's arrival, the medical missionary/surgeon was preparing to perform a very serious operation on a woman in a primitive, makeshift clinic. Still skeptical, his previous partner asked the missionary, "Do you remember how much money you would have made for just this one operation if you had performed it back in southern California?" The medical missionary replied, "Yes, I would have made several thousand dollars." His partner responded sarcastically by asking, "What will you make for it here?" The Christian surgeon quietly responded, "Well, there are several things I'll receive. First, if you look over into the next room, you will discover several children. Those children are the sons and daughters of the woman I'm about to operate on, and if she survives, I'll receive their thanks and love. Also, I if you look closely at the hand of the woman who is preparing for surgery, you will notice her fist is clenched. Inside that fist is a coin she wants to give to our mission clinic. It's a sacrificial gift of love. And, finally, there is one other thing I'll receive." The physician guest who had flown in to visit his friend asked, "What could that possibly be?" The missionary replied gently, "One 'well done, thou good and faithful servant' from my Lord Jesus Christ.'"

In Philippians 2:6-7, we read that Christ didn't think equality with the Father was a thing to be grasped, but instead he humbled himself, became a servant — and he called each of us to a life of service to others.

As a Christian seeking to grow spiritually, I have long believed that the central goal of my life is to be involved in a life-long process of becoming more like Christ (see Philippians 3:10, Romans 8:29, Colossians 1:27). If the goal of the Christian is to become more like Christ, then it is imperative for us to understand what Christ was truly like in his nature. While there are many places in scripture where we are told by others what Christ was like, there is only one place in all of the Bible where Christ himself tells us what he was like.

In Matthew 11:28, Jesus says, "I am gentle and humble in heart." The only time Christ described himself in all of the Gospel accounts, he tells us he was gentle and humble. Unfortunately, both of these terms — gentle and humble — have suffered through the centuries in terms of their essential meaning. The word "gentle" in the New Testament means "strength under control". A person who is growing spiritually in relationship to their Christ-like gentleness is one who develops an inner strength under the control of our loving God. The term "humble", in the context of New Testament Greek, means literally, "to stoop low as to serve." Accordingly, we may ask: Question - When am I most Christ-like? Answer - When I choose to live my life as a servant.

At the heart of our understanding of what it means to be growing spiritually is a heart-felt commitment to a life of service to others, beginning with our families. There is near universal agreement among centenarians that a pivotal characteristic in their pilgrimage toward reaching age 100 and beyond is the meaning and purpose they are finding in living lives of service to others.

There is one characteristic that I have frequently communicated to my children and grandchildren that they should expect to see in my life. The expectation they should have for their father and grandfather is that I am always seeking to be growing spiritually. I believe a crucial mark of healthy aging is a rejection of the concept that we ever reach a plateau where we begin to coast in our spiritual growth. Rick Warren writes wisely when he states, *"Spiritual maturity is neither instant nor automatic. It is a gradual, progressive process that will take the rest of our lives."*

Vital to my spiritual growth has been the commitment I made many years ago to be intentionally guided by four life practices that have sustained me through the years. I share these four spiritual disciplines with you as a love offering, knowing that these truths have served me well as I live out my spiritual life now in my eighth decade.

The First Life Principle

If we are to "grow young" and age in a healthy manner, we must accept ourselves as people of great worth and value in the sight of God.

Arthur Combs, for many years the head of The Department of Education at the University of Florida, along with a whole team of researchers, spent several years and over $100,000 researching one question: What are the ingredients that create a great teacher? They came to this conclusion: The top two ingredients of a great teacher are:

1. That the teacher will deeply love himself or herself
2. That the teacher will deeply love his or her students.

Thousands of dollars and years of research spent to conclude what scripture affirmed centuries ago. What is a mark of a person who is aging in a spiritually healthy fashion? A person who deeply loves himself or herself, and a person who deeply loves his family and friends.

As a Christian, I deeply believe that no matter what our appearance may be, no matter how intelligent we are, no matter how old we are, we are deeply, extravagantly, unconditionally, lavishly, radically, wildly loved by God — and accordingly we are to love ourselves.

Years ago, author Ed Farrell was visiting his uncle on his uncle's 80th birthday. Ed's uncle lived in Ireland, so Farrell flew from his home in the United States to be with his beloved relative, mentor and friend. Early in the morning on the first day of his visit, Ed's uncle climbed out of bed for his daily morning hike. As he circled around a scenic lake with his nephew, he whistled a happy tune. As he whistled, he would frequently break into a celebratory skip. At the midpoint of their hike, Ed asked, "Uncle, why has there always been so much joy in your life?" Ed's uncle quickly responded, "Oh, it's because of my Father! My heavenly Father! Oh, the Father — He is so fond of me!"

If we are to age in a healthy manner, we must accept ourselves as people of great worth and value in the sight of God, we must be able to affirm in our hearts, "Oh, the Heavenly Father! He is so fond of me!"

At the heart of our beings, many of us may have an identity crisis because we do not know who we are in God.

- A spiritually mature Christian believes in his heart that he is wildly, extravagantly, relentlessly, unconditionally loved by God.
- A spiritually mature Christian believes in his heart that he is "fearfully and wonderfully made" (Psalm 139:14) in the very image of God with unique gifts and talents.
- A spiritually mature Christian believes that when Jesus, The Good Shepherd, reaches out for His sheep to hold them in His gentle arms, He reaches out for us.
- A spiritually mature Christian believes in his heart that in the midst of a superficial culture that is trying at every turn to teach us that our worth is based upon our position, or title, or affluence, or appearance, that if we are stripped away of everything, we have tre-

mendous worth because we know who we are in the sight of God.

I believe that for those of us who are parents and grandparents that next to leading our children or grandchildren to Christ, the greatest legacy we leave is that we have given our children and grandchildren a vision as to who they are in God. Every morning, I seek to remind myself that I am a person of great worth and value in the sight of God.

The Second Life Principle

If we are to "grow young" and age in a healthy manner, we must accept full responsibility for our lives.

Psychologist Dr. Carl Rogers wrote wisely when he stated, "I know of only one type of person who will probably never become emotionally whole: the person who blames other people for his or her problems."

As you may know, there was a conventional psychological approach for several decades in this country which focused solely on analyzing our past — rather than placing an emphasis on present challenges and future responsibilities. The theory behind this past-centered approach was that by understanding all of the deprivation and hardships, influences and injuries of our past, we could gain insight into why we feel and act the way we do. Thus, we were able to blame others (parents, teachers, friends, a spouse, etc.) for causing all our present struggles. Calling this approach "the blame game", brilliant American psychologist Hobart Mowrer wrote, "The success of the blame game seemed complete. Only one thing went wrong — the patients did not get better."

Author John Powell, before his death, used to hang up a large sign on his bathroom mirror in order to protect himself from playing "the blame game". The sign contained the first words Powell would read every morning as he was shaving. In huge letters, the sign read: *"You are now looking at the face of the person who is responsible for your happiness today!"* One Christian psychologist put it this way, *"Growth begins when blaming ends."*

If we are to be growing spiritually through all the seasons of life, we must accept full responsibility for our lives.

The Third Life Principle

If we are to "grow young" and age in a healthy manner, we must continually decide to make our lives an act of love.

Dr. Elizabeth Kubler-Ross, renown psychiatrist and best-selling author of the book, *On Death and Dying*, told the story of a time when she was the head of staff for a group of psychiatrists on the East Coast who were seeking to minister to dying patients in a city hospital. Dr. Kubler-Ross became discouraged because she sensed that most of the professional psychiatrists were unable to truly break through and with empathy give hope and meaning to the terminally ill patients. At about the same time, Dr. Kubler-Ross began to observe that while a cleaning lady was working in each patient's room, she was able to inspire the dying men and women and offer them comfort and courage. Finally, Dr. Kubler-Ross approached the cleaning lady and tenderly asked her,

"What is your secret? How are you able to so impact our patients?" The cleaning lady responded quietly, "Oh, there is no secret. I just go into the hospital rooms, and I discover the patients are so afraid. I'm not afraid of death anymore. My little boy died of pneumonia when he was only three years old. So, whenever I feel led by God, I go up to these patients and I listen to them, and I hug them, and I love them."

Dr. Elizabeth Kubler-Ross immediately appointed this cleaning lady as her Assistant Head of Staff with oversight over all the psychiatrists in the hospital, much to their chagrin and dismay. Here was an uneducated Christian woman who had so yielded her life to the power of our loving God that she became a healing agent to hurting people. She had transformed her life into an act of love. Indeed, it is difficult to overstate the impact a person can have in life when that person consciously decides that, with the help of God, he or she will make his or her life an act of love.

In light of the theme of this book, it is important to

note that researchers are clearly demonstrating that men and women who choose to make their lives an act of love tend to live longer and healthier lives than the rest of the population. For example, Dr. Robert Butler and his colleagues at The National Institute of Health committed themselves to an eleven-year study following several hundred men and women between the ages of 65 and 95. They discovered that individuals who expressed a clear goal of serving others as an act of love tended to live an average of 7½ years longer than their peers, and continued to be significantly more mentally acute and protected from related illnesses such as diabetes, dementia and arthritis than their contemporaries. It appears that God has made us with an innate desire to love and serve — and that when we do, we tend to increase *both* our health span and our life span.

Over the past five decades, I have been invited to help a number of friends prepare for transitioning into a new season of life. My goal is always to help these men and women connect their spiritual gifts and talents with specific ministries that can better enable them to make their lives an act of love. In this regard, many have joined me in developing and refining a personal mission statement which focuses on such questions as:

- What am I passionate about in wanting to serve others?
- How can I best use my spiritual gifts and talents as I seek to make my life an act of love?
- What do I deeply love doing as I seek to intentionally serve others as an act of love?

When I turned 70, I revised my personal mission statement in the following areas:

1. I clarified my intentional strategies for serving and loving my family
2. I developed specific plans related to my writing two more books which I hope will encourage many others.
3. I listed specific ways that I could work to improve my speaking and teaching methodologies.
4. I made a renewed commitment to follow through on practical ways I can reach out to aging friends both locally and around the

country who are having difficulties transitioning into a new season of their lives.

5. I set concrete goals related to fund raising for Alzheimer's research.

6. I wrote out precise plans of action for deepening my relationships with each of my children, grandchildren, and with my close friends.

I commend to you the development of a personal mission statement. I have found it to be an extremely helpful process which hopefully serves as one component toward expanding my spiritual life.

One of my great heroes, theologian and medical missionary Albert Schweizer, wrote, "The only ones among you who will be truly happy are those who have sought and discovered how to serve others." Dr. Schweizer calls each of us to a life lived as an act of love.

The Fourth Life Principle

If we are to "grow young" and age in a healthy manner, we must live our lives as a great adventure.

Before his death, my friend and best-selling author Bruce Larson was given a seven-year grant by the Lilly Foundation to research only one question: What are the ingredients that can enable a person to live an emotionally healthy and fulfilling life?" Bruce interviewed pastors, psychologists and specialists from all over the world. He then came to this conclusion:

> *"The answers to my question implied that emotional wholeness varied considerably from culture to culture. Yet, after seven years of research, I did recognize that all of these experts agreed about one particular ingredient. They said, 'an emotionally and spiritually healthy person is someone who can choose a life of risk and adventure for a worthy cause."*

As Christians, we recognize there is no greater cause in life than to be a part of Christ's agenda in the world. Indeed, Christ affirmed centuries before Bruce Larson's research on this topic that "whoever would save his life will lose it, but whoever would lose his life for my sake will find it." (Matthew

16:25) Helen Keller stated it this way, "Life is either a daring adventure or it is nothing at all."

Years ago, a dear friend of mine had just completed his annual physical at the age of fifty. His physician, a wise Christian doctor, called my friend into his office, reviewed all his blood panels and other medical tests, and then said to him, "What you have is an attack of full-blown middle age. Middle age is a time when people are often advised to take it easy. You start to live very cautiously. You avoid anything new or risky. In so doing, you end up hastening the whole aging process."

Before her death, Mother Teresa wrote these wise words, "I used to pray that God would feed the hungry, but now I pray that He will guide me to do whatever I am supposed to do. I used to pray for answers, but now I'm praying for strength. I used to believe that prayer changes things, but now I know that first of all, prayer changes us — and we change things." Mother Teresa, right until her last day on earth, lived her life as a great adventure.

Sociologists tell us that one common factor found in

the five communities where the average life span is nearly 100 is this: "These villagers live their lives actively as a great adventure, continuing to work and serve and love their families and friends well into their late 90's." As mentioned previously in this book, these communities do not understand the concept of retirement. While we may retire from some career or vocation, we would be wise to never retire from asking the question, "What new adventure are you calling me to embark upon, loving God, in making a difference in your Kingdom agenda here on earth?" This process should never end until we pass into eternity.

When I pastored a wonderful congregation in Minneapolis many years ago, I invited onto my staff as Director of Singles Ministry a Christian woman named Diane Schmidt. At the age of 33, Diane developed a rare and aggressive type of esophageal cancer that had metastasized throughout her entire body. Weighing less than one hundred pounds, frail and often nauseated from her chemotherapy treatments, she called from Minnesota to my California home one evening. Diane shared with me that night that she had on her heart one last dream before her death: to travel to Forest Home Christian Conference Center located in the mountains of Southern California to spend her last days with our family. She had been to the scenic Forest Home campus once before, loved her time there, knew I was speaking there in August, and so she came. On the last evening of our week together there, we joined in a hymn sing beside a picturesque lake nestled in the mountains. As we drove back to our family cabin after singing some of the great hymns of faith, Diane said softly to me, "This has been one of the best days of my life." I responded, "Would you like to share your story of faith tonight to all the conference attendees before my teaching session?"

"Yes!" Diane immediately replied.

As Diane stood that evening weakened with her two hands holding up her body as she grasped the pulpit, she spoke to all in attendance about a "peace that passed understanding." The next morning, Diane had grown considerably weaker. I called for an ambulance to drive her down the mountain to a nearby hospital. She passed away later that day, but literally right until the very last day of her life, she chose to live life as a great adventure for Christ. So may we!

❖

Final Thoughts

"Tell me, what is it you plan to do with your one wild and precious life?"

Mary Oliver

"A joyful heart is good medicine."

Proverbs 17:22

Final Thoughts

THE ONE ATTITUDE CHOICE THAT IS CRUCIAL FOR HEALTHY AGING

Of the multitude of studies on healthy aging I have researched over the past three decades, I discovered one sociological study of particular interest. When a large number of centenarians were asked what they believed was the primary factor that enabled them to reach age 100 and beyond, they gave an answer surprising to the research team interviewing them. Far more often than these aging folks mentioned nutrition or exercise or any other factor, the men and women responded with a simple but profound answer. By an overwhelming margin, the number one reason the centenarians said they believed they had lived so long was an optimistic attitude toward life. Indeed, research does seem to suggest that undergirding the seven decisions I've reflected on in this book must be a daily positive attitude, rooted in gratitude.

Research indicates that while the habits of centenarians vary from country to country, the one characteristic they share in common is optimism. When difficult situations arise, whether it is the death of a loved one or illness that touches them personally, men and women who live to age 100 and beyond share a resiliency that enables them to stay positive. For example, a 2016 study of Ashkenazi Jewish centenarians concludes that optimism was the primary shared attitude of those who lived long and healthy lives.

Most of us as we age will tend to fall prey to one or more chronic diseases in mid to late life. This is also true of centenarians. The distinction that is important to note is that these folks appear to be remarkably resilient when it comes to shrugging off these ailments. The research is definitive! Living with optimism, kindness, gratitude and joy has tremendous positive consequences for our health and longevity.

Scientific research teaches us that our thoughts and emotions are in fact cellular signals that are involved in the process of translating information into physical reality. This close interaction between thought, emotion and bodily systems explains why recent widows are twice as likely to develop breast cancer, and why individuals who suffer from chronic depression are four times more likely to experience frequent illnesses. Clearly, negative thoughts have an impact on our physical health. However, there is an opposite and equally powerful upside.

For example, scientific research carried out at Duke University reported that in the 866 heart patients studied, those who routinely felt more positive emotions had a 20 percent greater likelihood of being alive 11 years later than the heart patients who experienced more negative emotions. A Johns Hopkins study reported that even in adults at risk of heart disease due to family history, a positive outlook offered the strongest protection against future congestive heart failure or cardiac arrest.

We recognize as we age that we are in charge of what we think. Further, we must understand that what we think will impact how our body responds to many illnesses. There is an irrefutable correlation between an optimistic attitude and longevity and radiant health. In the classic "Nun Study", researchers analyzed autobiographies from 180 Catholic nuns, written when the nuns were in their early 20's, and then followed the survival rate of the nuns decades later when these women were between the ages of 75 and 95. The nuns who expressed the most optimism, gratitude and other positive emotions lived as much as *ten years longer* than those with pessimistic and critical attitudes.

In a 2017 study, researchers at University College, London gauged the happiness levels of people ages 52 to 79 by monitoring their feelings several times over each day. Then, five years later, the researchers examined how many of these men and women had died. The result: older people who were optimistic had a 35% lower risk of dying over a five-year period than more pessimistic people. Even after the researchers factored in medical conditions including cancer and diabetes, being optimistic was still linked with living longer. Professor Andrew Steptoe, one of the study's researchers, noted, "I was surprised that optimism was such a strong factor in longevity even among people who had chronic diseases."

Robert Emmons, clinical psychologist and best-selling author, reveals in his extensive research the tremendous value of gratitude, which is closely linked to optimism, in relationship to health and longevity. Dr. Emmons states, "Grateful people have stronger immune systems, are sick less often, have lower inflammation levels, have lower blood pressure, and experience less depression and anxiety, all of which are strongly linked to greater longevity."

Optimism and gratitude support cardiovascular health as well as our immune systems, according to a study published in the American Journal of Cardiology. Further, a research paper released by the John Templeton Foundation showed that optimistic people have 10 percent fewer stress-related illnesses and tend to live up to seven years longer than those men and woman who test low on optimism.

One of my heroes, Dr. Martin Seligman, the pioneer of the positive psychology movement in the United States, and author of the book, *Learned Optimism*, provides us with perhaps the most extensive research on the impact of optimism. Seligman's research documents that optimists not only do better in the workplace and at school, but they also recover from setbacks more quickly and are less likely to battle depression. Of particular interest to me as I researched topics for this book was the reality that Dr. Seligman's extensive scientific studies revealed that optimists tend to be healthier, live longer and age better than their contemporaries.

Paralleling research referenced in *Learned Optimism*, a Mayo Clinic study that followed more than 800 people for 30 years discovered that optimists tend to live significantly longer than pessimists. Even after factoring age and sex into the results, the researchers found that the optimistic group's actual survival rate was significantly beyond the average life span, while the pessimistic group had a 19% increase in premature death. Further a survey of over 51,000 ethnically diverse Americans between the ages of 45 and 84 showed that optimists have amazing heart health. The men and women in this study who scored high on optimism were twice as likely to be in ideal cardiovascular health as compared to pessimists. Given that cardiovascular disease is the leading cause of death in the United States, a healthy heart is a significant contributor to longevity.

Of the myriad of studies available demonstrating the strong link between optimism and healthy aging, allow me to share one final research project. An analysis conducted by Yale University researchers asked people in their 50's or older to agree or disagree with statements such as:

- Do you think that things will get worse as you get older?
- Do you think you will become less useful as time goes by?
- Do you think you will be as happy as you were in your youth?

Twenty-three years later, it was discovered that people who viewed aging more positively lived an average of seven and a half years longer than those who perceived it more negatively. In this study, simply having an optimistic attitude made more of a difference in a person's longevity than did blood pressure, cholesterol levels, body weight, exercise or smoking.

In 2019, when I was diagnosed with prostate cancer, I had an attitude choice to make. Over the years, many of my friends have been diagnosed with various types of cancer. As I would meet and pray with them, some of my friends would say to me, "I'm not going to let cancer change me!" I understood the defiance and courage behind this statement. Yet for me, my daily prayer was, "*Loving God, change me through the experience of having cancer. Help me as I undergo months of treatment to become a better Christian, a better friend, a better father and grandfather. Help me to understand if there are decisions I can make that will enable me to be a better steward of my spiritual, emotional and physical health. Help me to live fully in the moment and experience the wonder of your creation each day. Finally, help me to make my life an act of love toward all those who care for me during my treatment sessions.*"

Looking back, I do believe that cancer changed me for the better. While I would prefer to not have to go through treatment for cancer again, I can candidly affirm that the experience was very positive and life-affirming. My radiology oncologist, Dr. Lindsay Blount, treated me as a whole person, not just a cancer patient. During our lengthy weekly sessions, we visited about not only my responsiveness to radiation treatment, but also about our families, running, weekend plans, movies, etc. He is such a true physician and became a friend. The radiology technicians, a wonderful group of young men and women at The Ridley Tree Cancer Center in Santa Barbara, brought joy and kindness to their daily interactions with me. When I would lay down to receive beam radiation therapy daily, a video of beautiful scenery would be played on the ceiling above me. Each day, one of the technicians would ask me what music I wanted to be played during my treatment. I asked for Roy Orbison so often that the team eventually didn't have to even wonder what my response would be. I could hear the amazing voice of "The Caruso of Rock" playing as I entered the treatment room. Occasionally when I left my daily session, I would be presented with a beautiful bouquet of flowers. I firmly believe that both the compassionate expertise of my treatment team and my optimistic attitude toward my daily sessions played a part in my recovery.

Today, as I continue to heal and recuperate, I renew each morning six commitments I have printed and attached to my bathroom mirror with the goal to honor them throughout the day. They are:

1. I accept total responsibility for my spiritual, emotional and physical health.

2. I am willing to adapt my lifestyle in any way that is beneficial to my health and longevity as new research emerges.

3. I am willing to take massive action to increase my health span and life span.

4. I will continue to make specific plans to fulfill my future dreams, goals and commitments I've made to serve others.

5. I will enjoy today as I seek to live in the moment with a heart of gratitude.

6. I will fully surrender my life today to God.

Years ago, I knew a middle-aged couple I'll call Bob and Mary. This married couple followed the majority of the many suggestions for healthy aging I have shared in this book. Tragically, Bob died suddenly of a massive heart attack in his 50's. Mary deeply loved her husband and grieved over his sudden death. Gradually, her grief led her into a season of prolonged depression. During this difficult time,

Mary stopped following the disciplined lifestyle she had once enjoyed with her life partner,

"Ron, Bob and I tried to live a spiritual, emotionally and physically healthy life, and look what happened to Bob! He's snatched away from me at such a young age." Over time, Mary began to isolate herself form her friends, stopped serving in her church, gained a significant amount of weight and stopped her once vigorous daily walks. I remember on one occasion visiting with Mary and gently sharing with her my beliefs about this one precious life we live.

"Mary, there are surely no guarantees in this fragile life we live. Our bodies are complex and there is no absolute certainty that we will live a long and vigorous life, no matter what choices we make. Yet, I've come to believe that even if it doesn't add one day to my life span, I want to live a life where I am building close bonds of love with family and friends. I yearn to live a life of meaningful service to others and to continue to challenge myself cognitively. I find joy in exercising in nature and eating in a healthy way. Peaceful sleep and a deeper walk with

God are important to me regardless of their potential impact on my life span."

As we shared together as friends over months of struggle and healing, gradually Mary chose to return to a lifestyle marked by the seven decisions in this book. She continues to this day to live a vital, vigorous and healthy life.

Our lives are just a gleam of time between two eternities — but God is at work in our lives to fan that gleam into a shining glory, the glory of His own reflected image. May we do our part each day to become all we are meant to be through all the seasons of our lives.

❖

RECOMMENDED READING

Of the scores of books I have read and researched over the past thirty years, I would highly recommend the following ten selections. I believe these ten books will be especially encouraging and insightful for you as we together seek to continue to "*Grow Young.*"

Love and Survival: Eight Pathways to Intimacy and Health by Dean Ornish, M.D.
Dr. Ornish, the pioneer physician who first demonstrated the link between diet and the reversal of heart disease, serves as President of The Preventative Medicine Institute in Sausalito, California.

Eat to Live by Joel Fuhrman, M.D.
Dr. Fuhrman serves as Director of Research for the Nutritional Research Foundation and is recognized worldwide as a leading advocate for a nutritarian, whole-food, plant-based diet.

The Blue Zones: Nine Lessons for Living Longer From the People Who've Lived the Longest by Dan Buettner.
Dan is an American National Geographic Fellow and

New York Times best-selling author. His 2009 TED talk on the topic *"How to Live to be 100"* has been viewed over four million times.

The Joy of Movement: How Exercise Helps us Find Happiness, Hope, Connection and Courage by Kelly McGonical, PhD.
Dr. McGonigal is a health psychologist and lecturer at Stanford University.

Healthy at 100 by John Robbins
Robbins was one of the first voices in the United States to demonstrate the link between nutritional and environmental concerns. He is a best-selling author and the founder of Food Revolution Network.

Why We Sleep: Unlocking the Power of Sleep by Matthew Walker, PhD.
Dr. Walker is a professor of Neuroscience and Psychology at the University of California, Berkeley.

Anti-Cancer Living: Transform Your Life and Health with the Mix of Six by Lorenzo Cohen, PhD.
Dr. Cohen serves as Director of Integrative Medicine, MD Anderson Cancer Center. He is also past President of the Society for Integrative Oncology.

Power Foods for the Brain by Neal Barnard, M.D.
Dr. Barnard is President of the Physicians Committee for Responsible Medicine and the best-selling author of 15 books.

How Not to Die: Discover the Foods Scientifically Proven to Prevent and Reserve Disease by Michael Gregor, M.D.
Dr. Gregor founded the website NutritionFacts.org in 2011 and is generally recognized as the leading researcher of the link between nutrition and health in the United States.

The Wounded Healer by Henri Nouwen. Nouwen was a Dutch Roman Catholic priest, author and theologian. He was a professor at the University of Notre Dame, Yale Divinity School and Harvard University. The author of 39 books, he concluded the final years of his life by serving special needs children at the L'Arche Daybreak Community in Richmond Hill, Ontario.

❖

ACKNOWLEDGMENTS

"Friendship has been the sheltering tree of my life."

Samuel Taylor Coleridge

From my initial research which started over thirty years ago, I have yearned for "Growing Young" to include scriptural insights, the most significant scientific studies related to healthy aging and a wide range of personal stories shared with me by family and friends. In this regard, the publication of "Growing Young" has been a synergy of input from scores of people I love.

My two children, Rachael and Nathan, have lovingly discussed with me all of the major concepts found in this book. They are my children, my friends, my confidants and my counselors. Their imprint is on every page of this book.

Rachael's and Nathan's life partners, Justin and Emily, have also been guides, encouragers, mentors and beloved friends to me for many years. I love them and they have helped me become a better person, parent and grandparent.

My four grandchildren, Caitlin, Griffin, Cami, and Griffin have brought great joy and meaning into my life. Their loving presence has enriched my life more than they will ever know. My relationship with each of them causes me to yearn to do my part in seeking to stay healthy, active, vital and available to them for hopefully many more years. An amazing joy that came into my life during the writing of this book was news from Nathan and Emily that they are expecting their first child — a girl! I can't wait to hold her and love her!

Stacy Madden is a long-time friend who has worked tirelessly alongside me in the development of "Growing Young". She has served in this project as my co-editor, graphic designer, typist and proofreader. Her deep Christian faith inspires me to seek to follow Christ more faithfully.

Joanne Bouslough has once again served in conjunction with Stacy as the co-editor of this book. Her wise counsel has been inspirational in my life and in the writings of my last three books. My close friends Dave Barry, Peggy Schierl, Kat Aker, Tim Thurman and Eva Cruz have all provided wise insights to "Growing Young". I will always be grateful for these special loved ones and their imprint on my life.

I'm grateful for the insightful essays that are shared in this book by my friends Don Nason, Bill Richardson, Gene Lucas and Dave Barry. I also deeply appreciate the permission of my friend Desirree Searl to share her inspirational story. A beloved group of friends have interacted with me as I have spoken on various topics addressed in this book. This community of companions include Ann and Rudy Aguilera, Mario and Claudia Morales, Charlie and Paula Johnson, Dave and Bonnie Schreiner, Roy and Cheryl Donkin, Dovie Schneider, Elaine Dodson, Gene Lucas, Jon Masuda, Sandie Miller, Greg and Nancy Johnson, Don and Judy Nason, Karen and Joe Fox, Dessiree Searl, Chuck Brown, Carol Brown, Gordon Azevedo, Barbara MacCullum, Larry and Carolyn Wilson, Jean Perrett, Janet Seaboyer, Jon and Shannon

McComb, David Marsango, Bob Mazawa, Bill and Mary Richardson and Yvonne Gilmore. Special thanks must be expressed to Bonnie Schreiner, whose initial input motivated me to write the concluding chapter of "Growing Young". Bonnie models the quality of optimism that exemplifies healthy aging.

Finally, I want to express my gratitude to you, the reader of this book. Many of you have also read other books I have written. Your thoughtful encouragement has motivated me to continue to research and to teach and to write. My prayer is that "Growing Young" will guide you to discover an even more vital, healthy and dynamic life lived in Christian service to others.

❖

Made in the USA
Monee, IL
04 November 2026

67377668R00108